Table o

Practice Test #1

Practice Questions

1. A healthcare quality management professional has all of the following responsibilities toward improving patient safety EXCEPT:
    a. Helping to develop a patient safety program
    b. Incorporating new technology into a patient safety program
    c. Setting and reviewing goals for a patient safety program
    d. Appointing a supervisor for a patient safety program

2. Which of the following types of charts is best for determining cause and effect?
    a. Control
    b. Fishbone
    c. Run
    d. Pareto

3. A hospital needs to decide whether or not to incorporate a new feature into its current services, and as a result has commissioned qualitative research that will provide detailed feedback. Specifically, the hospital would like to collect opinions from patients and other hospital customers with a wide range of experience and backgrounds. Which of the following types of assessments is most likely to be of use to the hospital?
    a. Survey
    b. Team analysis
    c. Focus group
    d. Case study

4. The process of risk management for the healthcare quality management professional includes all of the following EXCEPT:
    a. Identification of risk
    b. Analysis of effects
    c. Reporting of incidents
    d. Prevention of risk

5. A review of supplies determined that a clinic is running low on several items essential for operation. With recent budget cuts, the clinic has to review costs carefully to find the best price for each item. What is the healthcare quality management professional's role in this?
    a. Oversee the purchase of each item to ensure cost management
    b. Determine which items need to be purchased from which supplier
    c. Delegate the purchasing of each item to the appropriate department
    d. Assist in developing a list of suppliers, by cost, for each item

6. A hospital has implemented a quality program to improve the overall quality of patient care. It is discovered, however, that the program is running over budget, so the hospital administrative board conducts a review of the program to see if it should continue. What is the healthcare quality management professional's role in this?
    a. Prove to the administrative board that the quality program should continue in the hospital
    b. Assist the administrative board in making a final decision about the quality program
    c. Evaluate the financial benefits of the program and demonstrate these to the board
    d. Create a committee to review the quality program and develop a list of reasons to keep it

7. A hospital has found that the performance of one of its departments is consistently below the expected standards. The hospital administration wants to locate the source of the problems and see improvement in the department within six months. What is the healthcare quality management professional's role in this?
    a. Research the problems and develop a program that applies current standards to the department
    b. Recommend that the hospital replace the current administration of the individual department
    c. Advise that a performance improvement team be assembled to review and address the failings
    d. Review the expected standards and submit these to the department for immediate application

8. The administration of a hospital has discovered that a lack of communication among different hospital departments has led to overspending and unnecessary errors in patient care. The administration has asked the healthcare quality management professional to assemble a team that can improve department communication and address the problems. What type of team would be most useful for this task?
    a. Cross functional
    b. Work group
    c. Quality circle
    d. Self-directed

9. A clinic is looking into adding a new computer software program to update an outdated program. The new computer system will keep better track of patient records and will enable the clinic to streamline the care that patients receive. What is the healthcare quality management professional's role in this?
    a. Advise the clinic to implement the software because of its value in improving patient care
    b. Assist the clinic in evaluating the pros and cons of the software
    c. Research the history of the software to see how it has impacted other clinics
    d. Create a simulation for the software to allow the clinic to see how it operates day to day

10. All of the following represent federally-mandated patient rights in the United States EXCEPT:
    a. Right to informed consent for medical treatment
    b. Right to maintain the privacy of medical records
    c. Rights to obtain a copy of medical records
    d. Right to receive healthcare services

11. One of the largest departments within a hospital has been running over budget for some time. The increasing expenditure has become problematic, and therefore the department has been asked to maintain a budget. What is the healthcare quality management professional's role in this?
    a. Follow the hospital administration's guidelines in setting a budget for the department
    b. Provide the department with the software tools to enable it to set a manageable budget
    c. Appoint a financial advisor to support the department in developing a compliant budget
    d. Assist the department in developing a manageable budget and reviewing it for compliance

12. A hospital has recently conducted extensive updates on its website and wants to make sure that the new site is ready to be made available to the public. What is the healthcare quality management professional's role in this?
    a. Evaluate the changes that have been made in the website and recommend improvements
    b. Compare the website to other hospital sites to ensure that the new site compares favorably
    c. Review the website to ensure that the reported information is accurate and complete
    d. Compile a list of required information for the website and report this to the hospital

13. A disagreement has arisen between the hospital administration and the members of one of its departments. The disagreement is in connection with the authority of the different parties involved and whether or not the administration can require the department to perform a certain task. What is the healthcare quality management professional's role in this?
    a. Review the rules establishing authority and inform the parties about how these rules apply to the department and the administration
    b. Advise the department to respect the authority of the hospital administration and to follow its expectations for department performance
    c. Consider the statements from both sides and participate in finding a solution that meets the expectations of both parties
    d. Create a review board to act as a mediator between the hospital administration and the department to find an agreeable solution

14. To cut down on costs, a clinic has been hiring outside consultants to perform many of its tasks, but there are concerns that the performance of many of these consultants does not meet the state's standards for the clinic's operation. What is the healthcare quality management professional's role in this?
    a. Supply the consultants with the information about state standards and ensure full compliance
    b. Review the activities of the consultants and report the results to the clinic administration
    c. Create simulated activities to test the consultants and see if they are meeting the standards
    d. Develop educational programs to assist the consultants and ensure that the standards are met

15. Which of the following performance improvement models would be the best recommendation for a clinic that wants to discover the source of problems in patient care, eliminate these problems, and achieve consistently high quality results in patient care?
    a. FOCUS
    b. Six Sigma
    c. PDCA
    d. LEAN

- 6 -

16. All of the following are roles of the healthcare quality management professional in terms of performance improvement teams EXCEPT:
    a. Directing the activities of performance improvement teams
    b. Guiding the expectations of performance improvement teams
    c. Removing members from performance improvement teams
    d. Taking part as a member of performance improvement teams

17. After a performance improvement team has completed its activities, what is the primary role of the healthcare quality management professional?
    a. Disband the group and discontinue current activities of the performance improvement team but maintain a core group of members for ongoing review
    b. Compose and present a report to the administration about the results of a performance improvement team
    c. Disseminate the results of the performance improvement team to all employees within the health facility
    d. Report the performance improvement results to the public to ensure organizational transparency

18. A healthcare facility has decided to establish a performance improvement team to see where the facility can make positive changes. Before assembling the team, what is the primary role of the healthcare quality management professional in assisting the healthcare facility?
    a. Provide the healthcare facility with reports about performance improvement team results from other facilities to offer a comparison
    b. Research past performance improvement team results to see what changes can be made for the new team's activities
    c. Suggest appropriate members for the performance improvement team to ensure team unity and the completion of goals
    d. Aid in developing a list of performance standards for the performance improvement team to follow

19. A hospital's administrative board is interested in applying a national excellence model to its activities. What is the healthcare quality management professional's role in this?
    a. Research the available national excellence models and recommend the one to utilize
    b. Review various national excellence models and evaluate their applicability to the hospital
    c. Assemble a review team to consider the different national excellence models for the hospital
    d. Survey department activities to consider in conjunction with various national excellence models

20. Which of the following is the primary role of the healthcare quality management professional in terms of committee meetings?
    a. Lead the committee meeting as an objective participant
    b. Review the topics to be discussed in the committee meeting
    c. Organize and maintain the information from the committee meeting
    d. Disseminate information from the committee meeting to different departments

21. To assist with the process of organizational change, the healthcare quality management professional's role includes all of the following EXCEPT:
a. Providing information about organizational change to employees of the facility
b. Developing educational programs to enable the employees to understand the changes
c. Creating a written plan detailing the goals of organizational change
d. Dismissing employees who fail to follow the implemented changes

22. A healthcare facility would like to apply for an external quality award. The role of the healthcare quality management professional in this includes all of the following EXCEPT:
a. Reviewing the available awards to understand each of them better
b. Assisting in evaluating the different awards for relevance to the facility
c. Contributing to improving the facility's public image on its website
d. Ensuring that the facility's standards meet the requirements for the awards

23. Which of the following organizations is best known for its wide-ranging membership across the public and private sectors and its active approach to ensuring patient safety solutions in all healthcare facilities?
a. ICI
b. JCI
c. NQF
d. AMA

24. All of the following are useful performance improvement oversight groups for the healthcare quality management professional to recommend EXCEPT?
a. QM Committee
b. Self-Directed Committee
c. Steering Council
d. Quality Council

25. In a case of a customer complaint about a healthcare facility, the role of the healthcare quality management professional includes all of the following EXCEPT:
a. Analyzing the customer complaint
b. Suspending the staff member responsible for complaint
c. Reviewing staff behavior that contributed to the complaint
d. Creating customer surveys to avoid future complaints

26. A clinic is reviewing the option of adding a new program to its available treatments but needs to be sure the program is worth the cost. What is the first step that the healthcare quality management professional should take in this?
a. Create a cost-analysis plan that enables the clinic to add the program within budget
b. Revise the clinic's budget to ensure that the treatment program can be added
c. Contact other facilities to generate feedback and see if the program should be added
d. Research the program and submit information indicating the feasibility of adding it

27. A practitioner within a large hospital has committed a serious breach of protocol during treatment of a patient. The breach actually resulted in improving the patient's condition, and the practitioner is attempting to show that the standards fail to take all patient needs into account. What is the healthcare quality management professional's role in this?
    a. Study the practitioner's claims to revise and improve the current expected protocol
    b. Review the current protocol and assist in revising the case management plan if appropriate
    c. Submit to the practitioner the list of expected protocol and ensure it is followed
    d. Develop a disciplinary report that profiles the practitioner and ends incorrect treatment

28. To evaluate the activities of a performance improvement team, the healthcare quality management professional should do all of the following EXCEPT:
    a. Creating a training program for the performance improvement team
    b. Offering feedback to the members of a performance improvement team
    c. Analyzing the productivity reports from the performance improvement team
    d. Adding information from performance improvement teams into employee appraisals

29. A healthcare facility is conducting its annual employee evaluations and needs to collect information on the practitioners within the facility. What is the healthcare quality management professional's role in this?
    a. Interview each practitioner to make sure that current activities meet the standards
    b. Survey employees who work with the practitioners to ensure appropriate activities
    c. Create a list of standards to apply to the evaluation of each practitioner
    d. Assist in profiling practitioners and submitting this information to the evaluation process

30. A hospital would like to improve its patient safety outlook over the course of the next year. The role of the healthcare quality management professional in this situation includes all of the following EXCEPT:
    a. Assisting in developing a patient safety program
    b. Contributing to writing a plan for a patient safety program
    c. Enforcing the rules for a patient safety program
    d. Connecting the goals of the patient safety program with the larger goals of the organization

31. A hospital is undergoing a change in administration, and many employees feel that they no longer understand their expectations or the larger goals of the organization. The role of the healthcare quality management professional in this situation includes all of the following EXCEPT:
    a. Organizing committee meetings to review the changing policies of the facility
    b. Assisting in developing a clear list of strategic goals for the organization and its employees
    c. Developing a list of employee and administrative objectives to be met over time
    d. Participating in creating a mission statement for the new administration of the hospital

32. The results of a risk management project are completed, and a clinic now wants to ensure that the risk management is fully applied to avoid future problems. How might the healthcare quality management professional assist in this process?
    a. Create a list detailing the results of the risk management project and disseminate these to all employees for review
    b. Facilitate a performance improvement team to incorporate the risk management findings into the organizational goals
    c. Appoint an outside consultant to assist the clinic with risk prevention over the long term
    d. Develop a vision statement for the organization that addresses the need to prevent and avoid unnecessary risk

33. A healthcare facility has increased its focus on customer satisfaction and is interested in seeing how much of a difference there is (if any) between the goals of the facility and the actual response from customers that primarily include patients and their families. How might the healthcare quality management professional assist in this process?
   a. Contact staff members within each department to discuss their contribution to customer satisfaction
   b. Create a performance improvement team to focus on the task of improving satisfaction
   c. Allow employees within the facility to explain negative experiences with customers
   d. Create surveys that allow patients and their families to respond about their experience

34. A healthcare quality management professional is expected to contribute to the process of educating a facility's employees about patient safety goals. All of the following would fall within the expected process of education EXCEPT:
   a. Monthly reminder emails to the employees within each department
   b. Safety reminder documents posted in each department
   c. Education programs for patients to understand facility goals
   d. Occasional training events for employees to provide safety reminders

35. A healthcare facility has been very pleased with the results of the performance improvement teams that the healthcare quality management professional facilitated. Additionally, the facility has noticed that employee productivity has improved, and the facility would like to quantify this improvement. How might the healthcare quality management professional assist in this process?
   a. Develop a plan for adding the performance improvement findings and activities to employee evaluations
   b. Create a rewards hierarchy for each employee who participated in a performance improvement team
   c. Generate an annual bonus plan that provides an incentive to employees who participated on a performance improvement team
   d. Assist the facility in sending personalized messages to all employees who were part of a performance improvement team

36. A healthcare facility has committed to improving the overall quality of care for patients and their families during their stay at the facility. Among these goals in improved quality of care are the goal of increased safety, better nutrition, and staff friendliness. The role of the healthcare quality management professional in improving quality of care includes all of the following EXCEPT:
   a. Developing an educational program to help staff members interact appropriately with patients
   b. Providing each department of the facility with friendly reminders about patient safety
   c. Creating a disciplinary process for staff members who fail to treat patients in a friendly way
   d. Researching and providing the facility with different options to improve food choices

37. A hospital's official licensing is up for renewal, and without the renewal the hospital will have to cease all operations. What is the healthcare quality management professional's role in this?
   a. Communicating with the official licensing body to ensure that the renewal is completed
   b. Researching the licensing process to see if another licensing body would be a better option
   c. Completing all licensing documentation and submitting this in a timely manner
   d. Reminding all employees about the need to follow requirements for official licensing

38. A healthcare quality management professional's responsibility toward improving patient safety includes all of the following EXCEPT:
    a. Assisting in the development of a patient safety culture throughout the organization
    b. Researching technology options for improving the current patient safety program
    c. Incorporating patient safety goals into the governance documents of the organization
    d. Informing patients at the organization about the facility's patient safety goals

39. The standard policy at a hospital is that all patients who arrive at the emergency room with chest pains should immediately receive a dose of blood pressure medication and cholesterol medication. In recent weeks, a number of patients have objected to this, claiming that they have no diagnosed blood pressure or cholesterol problems and that the hospital should not give them medication without a clear diagnosis. A healthcare quality management professional's responsibility in this situation includes all of the following EXCEPT:
    a. Evaluate the practice of prescribing certain types of medication to emergency room patients regardless of diagnosis
    b. Communicate with other hospitals to see if they also follow a policy of prescribing certain medication to emergency room patients
    c. Review the current standards that created the practice of prescribing this medication under certain circumstances
    d. Compare the hospital's emergency room policy to current recommendations in the medical community

40. Following the implementation of large organizational change within a healthcare facility, what is the healthcare quality management professional's role?
    a. Facilitate educational programs to begin the process of implementing the change in the facility
    b. Survey patients to determine whether or not the change has improved the overall quality of care for them
    c. Consider whether the change has been effective and whether ongoing improvement needs to continue
    d. Assemble a performance improvement team to continue integrating the change within the organization

41. A recent review of the risk management process within a medical facility has revealed a number of serious failings. What is the healthcare quality management professional's role in preventing future risk management errors from occurring?
    a. Identify employees and staff members who contributed to the risk management failures
    b. Create a new risk management program that utilizes improvements in technology and identifies failures earlier
    c. Notify all employees about the risk management failures and disseminate information to prevent future failures
    d. Assist in revising the current risk management plan to take findings from the review into account

42. A healthcare facility has implemented a new patient safety program and has achieved positive results, notably improved performance among many employees and staff members. What is one appropriate way for the healthcare quality management professional may assist the facility after this successful outcome?
   a. Develop a reward program for employees and staff members who contributed to improving patient safety
   b. Provide informational opportunities to educate employees and staff members who did not contribute as much to the patient safety program
   c. Evaluate all employee and staff member activities with regard to how each has contributed to the patient safety program
   d. Apply the results of the program to employee and staff member evaluations to create a ranking system in the facility

43. A healthcare quality management professional's responsibility regarding information management in a healthcare facility generally includes all of the following EXCEPT:
   a. Define data
   b. Collect data
   c. Summarize data
   d. Qualify data

44. What is the healthcare quality management professional's primary role within a hospital that is seeking voluntary accreditation from a recognized accrediting body?
   a. Reviewing all recognized accrediting bodies to see what is available for voluntary accreditation
   b. Evaluating recognized accrediting bodies and assisting in selecting one appropriate for the hospital
   c. Recommending that best accrediting body for the hospital, taking the facility's specific situation into account
   d. Developing a presentation that provides all of the necessary information for selecting an accrediting body

45. A healthcare facility has just completed a year-long study to consider updates and improvements to be made within the facility. What is the next step that the healthcare quality management professional should take in this situation?
   a. Interpret the data from the study to support the decision-making process about applying updates and improvements
   b. Appoint an advisor to apply necessary updates and improvements from the study into the facility's activities
   c. Select which updates and improvements from the study to apply to the facility and which to reject
   d. Begin incorporating updates and improvements from the study into the facility's day-to-day activities

46. A significant clinical error has occurred during patient treatment, and as a result of this a regulatory body has been notified. What is the healthcare quality management professional's primary role in this situation?
   a. Review the regulatory body's standard rules and procedures that apply to this type of patient treatment
   b. Recommend the appropriate disciplinary action for the staff member or members involved
   c. Facilitate ongoing communication with the regulatory body to ensure a satisfactory solution
   d. Inform the healthcare facility about the steps that should be taken to avoid future errors

47. Following the results from a large-scale performance improvement study that has reviewed all departments of a healthcare facility, the healthcare quality management professional's primary role includes all of the following EXCEPT:
   a. Reviewing the results of the performance improvement study
   b. Applying the results of the performance improvement study
   c. Disseminating information about the study for employee education
   d. Evaluating the overall effectiveness of the performance improvement study

48. Regarding employee performance within a healthcare facility, the healthcare quality management professional's primary role includes all of the following EXCEPT:
   a. Assembling comparative data to measure employee performance
   b. Applying employee performance improvement to the facility's evaluation system
   c. Creating a program that recognizes employee performance improvement activities
   d. Identifying positive employee activity and indicating employees appropriate for promotion

49. Within statistical analysis, the "mean" might also be described as which of the following?
   a. Probability
   b. Average
   c. Dispersion
   d. Coefficient

50. Within statistical analysis, which of the following terms refers to the amount of variability from the mean?
   a. Expected average
   b. Causality expectation
   c. Standard deviation
   d. Observational error

51. Before the start of a performance improvement process, the healthcare quality management professional should do all of the following EXCEPT:
   a. Develop outcome measurements to determine the results of the performance improvement process
   b. Assist in developing projects for performance improvement teams to complete during the process
   c. Create educational opportunities for employees and staff members to learn about and apply performance improvement results
   d. Participate in establishing priorities for the activities that will occur during the performance improvement process

52. A practitioner decision has generated controversy within a healthcare facility. What is one important role of the healthcare quality management professional in this situation?
    a. Contact the regulatory body to determine the correct procedure for practitioner activities
    b. Interview staff members to determine whether or not a risk management review is needed
    c. Develop a performance improvement activity to ensure that facility procedure is followed
    d. Evaluate the evidence from the practitioner and compare it to current practice guidelines

53. Among statistical process control components, which of the following terms refers to an unpredictable or fluctuating value?
    a. Common variation
    b. Random variation
    c. Special cause variation
    d. Continuous variation

54. A healthcare facility that has a reputation for providing patients with consistently high-quality treatment has recently experienced problems with its computer system. The computer system has been malfunctioning, making it difficult for practitioners to access all of the details in patient records before treatment. The result has been several weeks of unusually sub-standard treatment for patients. Which of the following best describes this type of statistical variation for the healthcare facility?
    a. Common variation
    b. Random variation
    c. Special cause variation
    d. Continuous variation

55. A clinic has experienced a variety of problems due to unclear protocol regarding patient treatment. The result is that many patients have experienced excellent treatment, but a number have experienced unsatisfactory treatment. The disparity has resulted in complaints, and the clinic is determined to standardize the expectations for patient treatment to ensure high quality treatment for all patients who visit the clinic. What is the healthcare quality management professional's program role in this?
    a. Develop an educational program to inform each practitioner about the regulatory protocol for patient treatment
    b. Profile practitioners and study their activities to determine what has led to the disparity in patient treatment
    c. Participate in the development of clinical guidelines for practitioner response to patient conditions
    d. Create a performance improvement activity that informs patients about the changes that will be applied in the clinic

56. Which of the following best describes the statistical variation for the scenario presented in question 55, that of a clinic that offers widely varying treatment due to a lack of unclear protocol about patient treatment?
    a. Common variation
    b. Random variation
    c. Special cause variation
    d. Continuous variation

57. Regarding employee evaluations, the healthcare quality management professional is expected to do all of the following EXCEPT:
   a. Develop a ranking system that identifies which employees should be promoted and which should remain at their current grade
   b. Incorporate the findings from performance improvement activities into job appointment opportunities
   c. Identify improved employee activities and apply these activities to the facility's employee evaluation system
   d. Recognize employees who have contributed to performance improvement through a privilege delineation system

58. A large community clinic has given the healthcare quality management professional the task of creating a performance improvement plan for the records department. The clinic knows that the records department is in need of updates and improvements, but as the clinic survives entirely on public funding, there is increasing concern about the cost of the performance improvement plan. What is the appropriate response of the healthcare quality management professional is this situation?
   a. Develop a fundraising plan that provides the clinic with extra funds to conduct the performance improvement plan
   b. Create a budget and complete cost-analysis reviews throughout the performance improvement plan
   c. Review the clinic's overall budget and recommend cost-cutting measures for other departments
   d. Find opportunities to reduce costs and direct the performance improvement team to stay on budget

59. A healthcare quality management professional should typically maintain the confidentiality of all of the following performance improvement items EXCEPT:
   a. Results
   b. Activities
   c. Reports
   d. Records

60. A healthcare facility is making changes to its data collection system. What is the primary role of the healthcare quality management professional in this situation?
   a. Inform the healthcare facility about regulatory requirements for data collection
   b. Create a program that ensures the confidentiality of all data collected into the new system
   c. Assist in developing a methodology for different types of data collection
   d. Research data collection systems for the facility and ensure the new system meets the budget

61. A healthcare quality management professional has recently revamped a facility's patient safety program. All of the following represent essential follow-up activities EXCEPT:
   a. Informing patients about their rights, as provided by state and federal law
   b. Educating employees about the goals of the patient safety program
   c. Reviewing the patient safety goals periodically to ensure effective assimilation
   d. Developing opportunities to integrate patient safety goals into the facility

62. The healthcare quality management professional typically participates in all of the following processes EXCEPT:
    a. Medical record review
    b. Peer review
    c. Governance review
    d. Service specific review

63. Which of the following best expresses the way a healthcare quality management professional can utilize technology for a healthcare facility's patient safety program?
    a. Research available software and assist in selecting the best software option for the facility
    b. Work with the IT department to ensure that patient safety goals are met throughout the facility
    c. Send out email reminders about patient safety to each department within the facility
    d. Provide patient safety information on the facility's website for the public to review

64. The healthcare quality management professional should work to integrate performance improvements into all areas of a healthcare facility's governance EXCEPT:
    a. Bylaws
    b. Committee meetings
    c. Administrative policies
    d. Facility procedures

65. Following an audit by a regulatory body, what is the healthcare quality management professional's role in assisting a healthcare facility?
    a. Present the healthcare facility with the list of recommendations from the regulatory body
    b. Review the audits from the regulatory body and research improvements to be made
    c. Determine the source of the problems to ensure future compliance with regulations
    d. Integrate the recommendations of the regulatory body into the facility's goals and activities

66. A healthcare facility has asked the healthcare quality management professional to assist in the performance improvement process for the facility. All of the following are steps the healthcare quality management professional can take to get started on this process EXCEPT:
    a. Establishing strategic goals for the performance improvement teams
    b. Developing performance improvement activities for the facility to utilize
    c. Reviewing the performance improvement results for future application
    d. Creating projects for the performance improvement teams to complete

67. Which of the following awards, presented by the President, recognizes a healthcare facility for organizational excellence?
    a. Malcolm Baldridge Award
    b. NCHL Award
    c. Magnet Designation
    d. NQF Award

68. Which of the following awards recognizes a healthcare facility for excellence in nursing?
    a. Malcolm Baldridge Award
    b. NCHL Award
    c. Magnet Designation
    d. NQF Award

69. What is the primary role of the healthcare quality management professional in assisting a facility that hopes to receive a national healthcare quality award?
    a. Review the standards for the award and assist in evaluating the feasibility of applying for it
    b. Develop performance improvement teams to address any issues that might prevent application
    c. Contact the awards committees to understand the process and ensure application
    d. Compare the benchmarking data to ensure that the facility meets all of the requirements

70. A hospital has created controversy by allowing a popular fast-food chain to offer meals within the dining area. Objections have been raised about the decision, notably concerns about why the hospital would agree to allow food known for being unhealthy into a healthcare facility. Proponents of the decision have pointed out that the fast food chain also serves a number of healthy options, but there is little evidence that patients eating at the chain are making these healthy selections. What is the healthcare quality management professional's role in this situation?
    a. Assemble a performance improvement team to consider the impact of the decision and determine a future course of action
    b. Consider the evidence and offer the hospital guidance on making the best decision for the facility and its patients
    c. Review the hospital's contract with the fast food chain and see if there is any way to remove unhealthy menu options
    d. Research other fast food choices for the facility to ensure that patients have the best range of healthy food options

71. The supply department within a large healthcare facility has failed to order and deliver necessary supplies to another department. The supply department claims that it never received the order, but the department that placed the order is certain that the information was sent. What is the healthcare quality management professional's role in this situation?
    a. Appoint a new supply manager to ensure that the supply department receives all orders in a timely manner to provide the supplies
    b. Research the error that caused the breakdown in communications and develop a more effective process for supplies
    c. Assist the facility in clarifying the supply relationship between departments and review the process for ordering supplies
    d. Assess and recommend software programs that can improve the process for ordering supplies and avoid future errors

72. A clinic is interested in signing a contract with one of several large medical device firms to begin utilizing the firm's products in the facility. What is the healthcare quality management professional's role in this situation?
    a. Research the different firms and discover how effectively their support staff interacts with healthcare facilities
    b. Consider the ratings and safety history of each firm to ensure that the clinic makes the best contractual decision
    c. Facilitate all communication during the contract negotiation process and draw up the contractual agreement between the parties
    d. Support the clinic in determining and establishing the best contractual relationship with an external supplier

73. What is the primary role of the healthcare quality management professional in assessing and improving the quality culture within an organization?
   a. Create a survey program that allows staff members to comment on organizational errors that need to be corrected
   b. Review the various activities of the organization and develop a performance improvement program to apply changes
   c. Facilitate a focus group of patients to determine how well the organization is providing service and meeting patient needs
   d. Review the organization's website to ensure that all necessary information is conveyed to the public

74. Which of the following types of charts is best for indicating the most important factor in a large group of factors?
   a. Control
   b. Fishbone
   c. Run
   d. Pareto

75. Which of the following types of charts is used primarily to observe performance according to a set sequence of time?
   a. Control
   b. Fishbone
   c. Run
   d. Pareto

76. Which of the following types of charts is best for determining whether or not a process is stable?
   a. Control
   b. Fishbone
   c. Run
   d. Pareto

77. All of the following represent the primary ways that a healthcare quality management professional can link the performance improvement of a healthcare facility to its strategic goals EXCEPT:
   a. Identifying clear strategic goals for the healthcare facility
   b. Developing performance improvement activities to meet strategic goals
   c. Educating staff members about the strategic goals for the facility
   d. Informing patients about their legal rights, as provided within the facility

78. Which of the following represents an electronic entry process for physicians or practitioners to create patient treatment instructions?
   a. EMR
   b. BCMA
   c. CPOE
   d. JCI

79. Which of the following was designed for doctors and nurses to ensure that they are treating the correct patient with the correct medicine, at the correct dose, and to avoid any medical errors?
   a. EMR
   b. BCMA
   c. CPOE
   d. JCI

80. Which of the following represents a type of computerized patient record that is maintained within a local healthcare facility (and is typically not linked to other patient record systems)?
   a. EMR
   b. BCMA
   c. CPOE
   d. JCI

81. An incident report has revealed an error on the part of a practitioner's judgment within a clinic. What is the primary role of the healthcare quality management professional in this situation?
   a. Interpret the incident report and assist the clinic's administration in applying procedures to avoid future errors
   b. Note the error in the practitioner's profile within the clinic and apply it to the performance appraisal system
   c. Create a performance improvement project to educate the practitioner and prevent judgment errors in future activities
   d. Recommend a temporary suspension of the practitioner until the incident has been fully and satisfactorily resolved

82. What is the primary role of the healthcare quality management professional in considering benchmarking data?
   a. Researching the activities of other healthcare facilities to ensure that the facility is meeting all expected standards
   b. Developing a marketing campaign to indicate to potential patients and/or customers why the facility is the best choice
   c. Facilitating performance improvement projects to make positive changes and keep the facility comparable to others
   d. Reviewing the healthcare facility's performance and comparing this performance to other facilities in the same class

83. All of the following indicate the role of the healthcare quality management professional for the upcoming licensure of a facility EXCEPT:
   a. Reviewing all licensure expectations and presenting any necessary improvements to the facility
   b. Evaluating the effectiveness of performance improvement training projects in the facility
   c. Preparing appropriate survey preparation training to ensure satisfactory licensure of the facility
   d. Developing and facilitating educational opportunities for staff members to understand licensure

84. Which of the following types of statistical analysis might be used to compare the results of people trying out a certain type of new medication against those in the placebo group?
    A. Regression analysis
    B. Probability analysis
    C. T-test analysis
    D. Parametric analysis

85. Which of the following types of statistical analyses might be used to determine the success rate of a recommended health regime against the independent variables of each patient's background and lifestyle?
    a. Regression analysis
    b. Probability analysis
    c. T-test analysis
    d. Parametric analysis

86. Which of the following represents the first step that the healthcare quality management professional should take before assembling a performance improvement team?
    a. Collect organizational data for analysis
    b. Identify patient safety goals to apply
    c. Communicate with an accreditation body
    d. Survey customers for needed improvements

87. The healthcare quality management professional can expect to contribute to the development of survey processes for all of the following EXCEPT:
    a. Accreditation
    b. Safety policy
    c. Governance
    d. Licensure

88. To assist with meeting the operational goals of a facility, the healthcare quality management professional should contribute to a written plan for all of the following EXCEPT:
    a. Care management
    b. Disease management
    c. Case management
    d. Practitioner management

89. In terms of performance measurements, which of the following represents a way to connect the activities of an organization to its larger strategies?
    a. Dashboard
    b. Balanced Scorecard
    c. Quality Management
    d. Core Measures

90. In terms of performance measurements, which of the following represents a collection of all performance data from within an organization?
    a. Dashboard
    b. Balanced Scorecard
    c. Quality Management
    d. Core Measures

91. In terms of performance measurements, which of the following is derived from a national performance system developed by Joint Commission?
    a. Dashboard
    b. Balanced Scorecard
    c. Quality Management
    d. Core Measures

92. What is the primary role of the healthcare quality management professional regarding the integration of quality concepts within an organization?
    a. Creating training programs that inform staff members about the organization's quality concepts and the expectations for them
    b. Reviewing benchmarking data from other facilities to ensure that all standards are being met within the organization
    c. Defining the quality concepts for the organization and developing ways to incorporate these concepts into day-to-day activities
    d. Incorporating quality concepts into the employee appraisal system to reward employees who effectively apply the concepts

93. Regarding the different types of data that apply to an organization, the role of the healthcare quality management professional includes all of the following EXCEPT:
    a. Delegating
    b. Collecting
    c. Defining
    d. Summarizing

94. Research has indicated that which of the following has the biggest effect on the failure of an organization to correctly apply medical ethics to patients?
    a. Inadequate training of staff members
    b. Breakdown of communication within the facility
    c. Unclear information about legal requirements
    d. Inconsistency between state and federal expectations

95. The healthcare quality management professional's responsibility toward risk management includes all of the following EXCEPT:
    a. Ongoing collaboration with the quality department
    b. Analysis of any failure that has occurred
    c. Assistance in review of medical records
    d. Coordination of risk prevention activities

96. Which of the following indicates one primary responsibility of the healthcare quality management professional in linking risk management with a facility's overall performance improvement goals?
    a. Complete a risk management assessment, and integrate this assessment with performance improvement activities for the facility
    b. Detail risk prevention activities for the facility, and identify opportunities for updating or redefining performance improvement goals
    c. Review the major causes of risk within the facility, and develop a performance improvement program to reduce or eliminate them.
    d. Assemble a performance improvement team to address potential risk within the facility and present the administration with recommended changes

97. Risk management as applied to a patient safety program should focus primarily on all of the following EXCEPT:
   a. Analysis of the root cause of the failure
   b. Review of the incident report detailing the failure
   c. Evaluation of the event that triggered the failure
   d. Application of patient advocacy laws to avoid future failure

98. A department within a healthcare facility has been criticized for failing to follow all of the required procedural steps in patient care. The department has argued that a number of steps are unnecessary and only slow down the process, reducing the quality of patient care. The facility has responded that the procedural steps are there for a reason, that the department is responsible for following the rules. What is the role of the healthcare quality management professional in this situation?
   a. Develop a review committee that takes the department's claims into consideration and compares their results against the procedures
   b. Facilitate ongoing communication between the department and the administration and participate in a careful review of the procedures
   c. Devise a performance improvement activity that enables the department to follow the procedures without sacrificing the quality of patient care
   d. Review the current procedures to determine if items are outdated or need updating, and consider applying procedural changes to patient care

99. Clashes have arisen between the supervisor of a department in a healthcare facility and the employees of that supervisor. The supervisor claims that the employees are not behaving respectfully, that work is not being completed within the required timeframe, and that the employees are now going out of their way to perform poorly and make her look bad. The employees claim that the supervisor treats the employees with little respect, that the timeframes are unreasonable, and that the supervisor looks for opportunities to criticize employee work to boost the image of her own credibility as a leader. What is the best response from the healthcare quality management professional in this situation?
   a. Mediate a discussion between the supervisor and the employees to ensure that each side has a fair say talking about the problems that have arisen
   b. Submit to the employees a reminder about the lines of authority within the facility and ensure that the supervisor is treated with respect in the future
   c. Recommend that the facility consider moving the supervisor to a new department and bringing in someone with whom the employees can work
   d. Develop a performance improvement program that will educate each side about its roles and establish an effective working relationship in the department

100. A good vision statement for a healthcare facility should contain all of the following EXCEPT:
   a. A definition of the expected outcomes
   b. A discussion of operational goals
   c. A statement about intended profits
   d. A personalized approach to an image

101. A department within a clinic has ended a long-term relationship with a supplier due to an increasingly poor quality of the supplies that were purchased. But the department is also running low on inventory and needs to find a new supplier to meet its needs. What is the primary role of the healthcare quality management professional in this situation?
    a. Research, identify, and recommend the best supplier for the department's needs
    b. Draw up the documentation that formally ends the relationship between the department and the supplier
    c. Create a list of potential suppliers for the department administration to review
    d. Evaluate all suppliers whom the department is considering and review contract expectations

102. A healthcare facility is facing criticism for inadequate patient treatment, and upon looking into the matter further a review board discovers that most of the problems are related to the equipment that is being used. In particular, the equipment is poorly maintained and thus is inconsistent in how it functions: on some days, the readings are accurate, while on other days the readings prove to be highly inaccurate. Which of the following best describes this type of statistical variation for the healthcare facility?
    a. Common variation
    b. Random variation
    c. Special cause variation
    d. Continuous variation

103. A small community clinic has been working hard to provide affordable healthcare to low-income families, but the clinic receives very little funding of its own. Because of this, staff members are in an outdated facility with poor ventilation, bad lighting, and faulty wiring. The doctors and nurses do their best to provide high quality patient care, but the results often reflect the low quality of the facility's condition. Which of the following best describes the type of statistical variation that occurs in patient care at this location?
    a. Common variation
    b. Random variation
    c. Special cause variation
    d. Continuous variation

104. A number of patients who received pacemakers at a hospital have complained that instead of feeling better, they feel worse. They have low energy and find themselves needing to rest for long periods of time after completing only a small task. Upon looking into this further, it is discovered that the patients' doctor has completely failed to adjust the settings according to patient needs. Instead, he simply gave each patient a pacemaker with the factory settings. Once the pacemakers have been adjusted to fit individual patient requirements, patients returned to say that they have been feeling great and have more energy than ever. Which of the following best describes this type of statistical variation among patients?
    a. Common variation
    b. Random variation
    c. Special cause variation
    d. Continuous variation

105. A tornado has veered off the expected course and has passed through a community. The area healthcare facility has lost power in several departments. The facility is struggling to activate its generators, but there are concerns that patient needs cannot be met. Which of the following best describes this type of statistical variation for the healthcare facility?
  a. Common variation
  b. Random variation
  c. Special cause variation
  d. Continuous variation

106. A healthcare quality management professional is reviewing patient information during an officially approved experimental treatment. Which of the following reflects qualitative data among the patient details?
  a. Blood pressure readings
  b. Changes in weight
  c. Mood during treatment
  d. Cholesterol levels

107. A healthcare quality management professional is reviewing the activities of a department within a healthcare facility. Which of the following does NOT reflect quantitative data in reviewing the department's information?
  a. Paper records maintained by the department
  b. Behavior of employees to customers
  c. Average hours worked by each employee
  d. Productivity rate of department

108. Two departments within a hospital share responsibilities for patient treatment. The hospital administration decided to make some changes, with the result that one of the departments is now responsible for the majority of patient treatment. During the course of the change, several of the patients failed to receive important parts of the treatment, and the two departments are now at odds with one another; the department taking over most of the treatment claims that the change was not fully completed, and that therefore the other department still had responsibilities. The other department disagreed. What is the role of the healthcare quality management professional in this situation?
  a. Present to each department the information about its current responsibilities to prevent future problems
  b. Mediate between the departments to ensure a clear understanding of roles and follow up with patients about treatment
  c. Cite the departments for failure to complete patient treatment and recommend further disciplinary action be taken
  d. Communicate with patients to explain the cause of the error and work privately with them to avoid legal action

109. A department within a healthcare facility has consistently been going over-budget. The department claims that its budget is not sufficient for its required activities, while the facility claims that the department is spending excessively and needs to reduce costs. What is the role of the healthcare quality management professional in this situation?
  a. Assist the department in setting up a manageable budget and working within it
  b. Communicate between the department and the facility to ensure a satisfactory agreement
  c. Establish for the department a clear budget that reflects the facility's expectations
  d. Review the activities of the department to see whether there is anywhere to cut costs

110. A large clinic is looking to introduce some costly changes into the facility. These changes will require careful budgeting. The healthcare quality management professional is likely to assist the facility in all of the following EXCEPT:
    a. Reviewing staff salaries to cut unnecessary expenses on benefits programs
    b. Supporting the facility in setting up a budget for effecting the changes
    c. Providing a cost analysis of the changes to ensure a satisfactory cost-return ratio
    d. Researching potentially unexpected costs to avoid going over-budget

111. All of the following represent essential performance improvement measures within a healthcare facility EXCEPT:
    a. Evaluating productivity of employee activities against established standards
    b. Reviewing the effectiveness of technology that is applied within the facility
    c. Utilizing historical data to consider the current outcome patterns of the facility
    d. Comparing the performance of the facility to that of similar facilities

112. A large hospital offers limited times during the day when family members are allowed to visits patients in the ICU. These limited times are strictly enforced, and even family members who are a couple of minutes late are sent away from visiting the ICU. The result is that customers are now complaining about the lack of available visiting times, as well as the inflexible standards. What is the primary role of the healthcare quality management professional in this situation?
    a. Review the current visiting times and encourage the facility to provide extended visiting times for family members
    b. Provide a communication process whereby family members can file formal complaints about the situation
    c. Submit to all family members a copy of the hospital's policy regarding ICU visits and explain the reasoning for it
    d. Assist the hospital in responding to customer complaints and review options for integrating a new policy

113. A large healthcare facility is looking into adding a new computerized system for collecting patient data. What is the primary role of the healthcare quality management professional in this situation?
    a. Research available systems and assist the facility in evaluating and choosing the best system
    b. Review all data collection systems to select the most effective one for the facility's needs
    c. Consider the details of all available systems to ensure the selected one meets all standards
    d. Submit a recommendation for the best computerized data collection system to the facility

114. Which of the following best describes the purpose and value of a scattergram chart?
    a. To compare two different variables of data
    b. To consider a change in data over time
    c. To indicate the probability of change in data
    d. To specify the proportion of each variable

115. A performance improvement plan should include all of the following EXCEPT:
    a. A defined list of priorities among the performance improvement activities
    b. Comparative research of external performance improvement plans
    c. A clear definition of the performance problem that needs to be addressed
    d. An established list of standards to be met during performance improvement

116. Which of the following best represents the goal of a healthcare facility in maintaining organizational transparency for the public?
    a. Complete public availability of all records that are not protected by privacy laws
    b. Full presentation of facility goals, objectives, and standards on the public website
    c. Public accountability for all facility leadership when mistakes occur within the facility
    d. Active leadership to ensure the public image matches the private one as closely as possible

117. All of the following are important elements of organizational transparency for a healthcare facility EXCEPT:
    a. Annual reports about facility costs and activities
    b. A public statement about facility values
    c. A public explanation of all activities within facility
    d. Clear information about facility partnerships

118. Which of the following best defines by-laws for a healthcare facility?
    a. A list of state and federal requirements by which the organization is expected to operate
    b. A list of legal conditions for patient treatment and practitioner activity within the facility
    c. A list of patient rights and ethics which govern all employee practices within the facility
    d. A list of organizational laws that define activities and procedures within the facility

119. Which of the following best defines utilization management?
    a. Assessment of various healthcare services based on whether they are necessary and efficient
    b. Internal review of facility procedures based on federal legal standards for facility operation
    c. Self-review of facility activities by a licensed group of experienced professionals
    d. Measurement of facility performance to ensure that it meets all internal and external standards

120. The techniques of utilization management include all of the following EXCEPT:
    a. Case management
    b. Demand management
    c. Peer review
    d. Disease management

121. What is the primary role of the healthcare quality management professional in terms of consultant activity within a healthcare facility?
    a. Monitoring all consultant activity to ensure that it meets the standards for quality and patient safety
    b. Researching the history of consultant activity by contacting other facilities and requesting information
    c. Communicating to the consultant all information about facility expectations for patient treatment
    d. Assembling a review team to ensure that the consultant follows facility procedures and policies

122. Which of the following types of team structures is best for a project that requires a measure of autonomy and can complete tasks with limited oversight?
    a. Cross-functional
    b. Work group
    c. Quality circle
    d. Self-directed

123. Which of the following types of team structures is best for combining employees with different skill sets and areas of experience to complete a task?
   a. Cross-functional
   b. Work group
   c. Quality circle
   d. Self-directed

124. All of the following reflect important qualities of effective teams EXCEPT:
   a. A solid sense of goals and responsibilities for the team
   b. A clear leader to guide the activities of the team members
   c. Good internal relationships among the members of the team
   d. A willingness to discuss the effectiveness of decisions and activities

125. A healthcare quality management professional has been given the task of assembling a performance improvement team. In selecting member of this team, he should focus primarily on all of the following EXCEPT:
   a. The previous experience of the employee in team activities
   b. The personal strengths and skill sets of each employee
   c. The effective problem-solving abilities of the employee
   d. The ability of the employee to listen and contribute

Answers and Explanations

1. D: In terms of improving patient safety, the healthcare quality management professional's responsibilities include the following: helping to develop a patient safety program, incorporating new technology into a patient safety program, and setting and reviewing goals for a patient safety program. The healthcare quality management professional's responsibilities do not necessarily include the responsibility of appointing a supervisor for a patient safety program. That particular task will likely fall to others within hospital administration.

2. B: A fishbone chart is most useful for helping to determine cause and effect. A control chart is useful for seeing the changes in a process; this would include effects but not necessarily causes. A run chart is most useful for viewing data over a time sequence. A Pareto chart uses two types of charting techniques to determine statistical information, but it is not necessarily useful for determining cause and effect.

3. C: The focus group will be most useful in providing the hospital with a broad range of opinions, as well as detailed feedback. The survey would limit answers to those available among the answer choice options, so this would not necessarily guarantee detailed feedback. The team analysis would largely remove patient and customer opinion from the decision. The case study would isolate findings to a single scenario and would fail to offer broad findings and detailed feedback.

4. C: The healthcare quality management professional is responsible for the following, in terms of risk management: identifying the risk, analyzing the effects of the risk, and preventing the risk. These responsibilities do not necessarily include the responsibility of reporting an incident of risk; that may or may not apply, depending on the source of the risk. (It should be noted, however, that the healthcare quality management professional is responsible for reviewing the incident report about the risk; of course, this is not the same as actually reporting an incident of risk.)

5. D: Among the answer choices provided, the healthcare quality management professional is responsible only for assisting in the process of developing a list of suppliers. The responsibilities do not include overseeing the actual purchase (as this is the responsibility of the purchasing department), determining the specific items (as this falls to individual departments), or delegating the purchasing of each item to the appropriate department (as most large purchases would be grouped under the responsibility of the purchasing department).

6. C: The role of the healthcare quality management professional is to evaluate the financial benefits of the quality program and to present these to the board. The healthcare quality management professional is not obligated to prove to the board that the quality program should continue; indeed, unless asked specifically to do so, this would be overstepping the boundaries of professionalism. He also is unlikely to assist the board in making a final decision or creating a committee to review the program. Again, unless the healthcare quality management professional is asked to perform any of these tasks, the role is limited to one of evaluating the financial benefits and demonstrating them as objectively as possible.

7. C: The primary role of the healthcare quality management professional is this particular situation is to advise the assemblage of a performance improvement team that can review and address the failings. The healthcare quality management professional might be involved in researching the problems, but the development of a program that applies the standards to the department would exceed his responsibilities. He would certainly not be expected to advise the hospital to replace the

current administration of the department; this would be the role of a larger group (such as a performance improvement team) that takes the time to review the situation. Also, he would need to do far more than simply submit the expected standards to the department for application. Obviously, the department is already failing to apply the standards, so something more needs to be done.

8. A: The key here is the need for a team that can find ways to improve communication among the different departments. This type of team would need to be cross functional, because it would be composed of people from the different departments who would then be delegated to communicate with one another and pass on the communication to others in their respective departments. The other types of teams – work group, quality circle, and self-directed – all have their place in professional improvement, but a cross-functional team would be best in this situation.

9. B: In this situation, the healthcare quality management professional's role is limited primarily to assisting the clinic in evaluating the pros and cons of the software. Advising the clinic to adopt the software would come after the necessary evaluation process, while researching the software and creating a simulation would be part of the evaluation process, but each item is limited in itself. The larger goal for the healthcare quality management professional is one of evaluation to assist the facility in making the best decision.

10. D: There is no federally mandated right to healthcare services for people in the United States. There are other statutes – such as the law that forbids emergency rooms from turning away people without insurance – but the federal government does not guarantee to people that they have the right to receive healthcare services. The other rights listed (right to informed consent, right to privacy, right to a copy of medical records) are all protected at the federal level.

11. D: The healthcare quality management professional is responsible for assisting the department in developing a manageable budget and reviewing it for compliance. He or she is not necessarily responsible for setting the budget; that would require the assistance of the department. Providing software tools to help with developing a budget would be part of the process, but the process is not limited to this. Additionally, the healthcare quality management professional might appoint a financial advisor, but this again is part of the process but not the only part.

12. C: In terms of public reporting, such as websites, the healthcare quality management professional's role is primarily one of ensuring that the information presented to the public is accurate and complete. He might evaluate the changes and recommend improvements, but this falls under the larger role of making sure the information is accurate and complete. Similarly, the other answer choices – comparing the new site to other hospital sites and compiling a list of required information – would fall under this larger category of ensuring accuracy and completeness in the information.

13. A: In terms of a dispute, the healthcare quality management professional's role is only to understand how the lines of authority are drawn and to present this information to the parties involved. He should not take sides in any way, making answer choice B incorrect. Additionally, he is not responsible for mediating or even finding a solution (unless asked specifically to do so). The role in this case is largely one of providing the information and allowing the parties to consider it.

14. B: The healthcare quality management professional is not responsible for overseeing consultants in general, but in the case of a failure in consultant activities, he or she is expected to review the activities of consultants and report on results. Answer choices A, C, and D all contain

- 29 -

details that might be part of the review process for the healthcare quality management professional, but they lack the larger role of reviewing and reporting.

15. B: Six Sigma is recommended as a performance improvement model that enables an organization to reduce problems and, more importantly, achieve consistency in results. The other performance improvement models – FOCUS, PDCA, and LEAN – offer variations of problem identification and reduction, but only Six Sigma specifically focuses on generating consistently good results.

16. C: The healthcare quality management professional is not necessarily responsible for removing members from the performance improvement teams. He might recommend removal, but the decision is likely to come from a higher source. The healthcare quality management professional is, however, expected to direct the activities, guide the expectations, and take part as a member of performance improvement teams.

17. B: After a performance improvement team has completed its activities, the healthcare quality management professional is expected to compose a report and present the results to the healthcare facility's administration. The healthcare quality management professional does not necessarily have the authority either to disband the team or to maintain a core group for ongoing review. He is also unlikely to disseminate the results to other employees; the purpose of the performance improvement team is generally intended for administrative review. Also, unless the public has been made aware of the performance improvement team, there is no need to report the results to those outside the facility.

18. D: Before the team is assembled, the primary role of the healthcare quality management professional is to aid the facility in developing a list of performance standards for the team to follow. After all, the team cannot accomplish much if it does not know what the goals are. The other answer choices represent activities that might be part of the process, but the primary step is certainly to identify the standards.

19. B: In terms of national excellence models, the healthcare quality management professional should review the different models and evaluate their applicability. He does not necessarily have the authority to recommend one in particular; the goal is more one of providing the facility with the information it needs to make a decision, and the decision itself is likely to come from a group of people. The healthcare quality management professional does not need to assemble a review team; he should already be somewhat familiar with the different models and should be able to generate an evaluation without the assistance of a review team. Finally, he does not need to survey department activities, as it is likely that these are already familiar.

20. C: For committee meetings, the healthcare quality management professional should be involved in organizing and maintaining the information from the meetings; this information might include the minutes from the meetings or any reports presented at the meetings. The healthcare quality management professional does not need to lead the meetings or disseminate information from meetings to the departments. It should also be noted that the activity of reviewing topics from the meeting is likely to fall under the larger role of organizing and maintaining meeting information.

21. D: It is not the responsibility of a healthcare quality management professional to dismiss any employees, with the possible exception of employees who fall under him specifically. The healthcare quality management professional is, however, responsible for providing employees of the facility information about organizational change, developing educational programs that enable

the employees to understand the change, and creating a written plan detailing the goals of the organizational change.

22. C: Regarding an external quality award, the healthcare quality management professional has several responsibilities. Among these might be the responsibility to review the available awards to ensure that each is fully understood (thus avoiding unnecessary application), to assist in evaluating the awards for applicability to the facility, and to ensure that the facility meets all of the standards for application. A campaign to improve the facility's public image on its website is not necessarily part of this process and might appear to be disingenuous and work against the facility's chances of receiving the award.

23. C: The NQF, or National Qualify Forum, is known for its wide-ranging membership across the public and private sectors and its active approach to ensuring patient safety solutions in all healthcare facilities. (The key in this question is the statement about "public and private sectors," since that sets the NQF apart from other patient safety organizations.) Answer choices A, B, and D include other organizations that focus on patient safety (among other things) – the ICI, the JCI, and the AMA – but none meet the specific description in the question.

24. B: Useful performance improvement oversight groups include the QM Committee, Steering Council, and the Quality Council. The Self-Directed Committee does not really exist, as the idea of being "self-directed" reflects more a type of team to apply in the workplace.

25. B: The healthcare quality management professional does not usually have the authority to suspend a staff member responsible for causing a customer complaint. (He may recommend a suspension, but the decision to suspend will come from another source.) On the other hand, the healthcare quality management professional is obligated to analyze a customer complaint, review staff behavior that contributed to the complaint, and create customer surveys to avoid situations leading to future complaints.

26. D: In terms of cost-analysis for a program, the healthcare quality management professional's first step is one of evaluating the feasibility of it. At some point, he might also create a cost-analysis plan that enables the clinic to add the program. He might also submit budget revisions that make the program possible and/or contact other facilities for feedback about similar programs. The first step, however, is simply that of evaluation: is the cost-return ratio feasible?

27. B: When a practitioner breaches protocol, the healthcare quality management professional is somewhat peripheral. That is to say, he should review the protocol that exists and determine if the case management plan for similar situations should be revised. Answer choice A says something similar, but the assumption in this option is that the practitioner's decision should necessitate a change in protocol. This may or may not be the case, so the situation should first be reviewed. Answer choice B assumes that the facility is ignoring the information from the practitioner and overriding the need for any changes; once again, a review should precede this. Answer choice D involves the healthcare quality management professional directly in the situation, and this would be incorrect.

28. A: Question 28 assumes that the performance improvement team already exists and is active in the process of performance improvement. Thus, the training program would be ex post facto at this point. The healthcare quality management professional should, however, offer feedback to the members of the team (to assist them in continuing the process), analyze the productivity reports from the team, and add information from the team into employee appraisals.

29. D: Once again, the healthcare quality management professional's role is somewhat peripheral: he should focus on profiling the practitioners and submitting the information to the evaluation process. It is not necessary – and is more likely to be inappropriate – for him to question the practitioners directly about their activities or to survey employees about practitioner activities. Additionally, the list of standards is already likely to have been created as part of the evaluation process, so there would be no need to do so at this point.

30. C: Regarding a patient safety program, the healthcare quality management professional has the following responsibilities: assisting in developing the patient safety program, contributing to a written plan for it, and connecting the goals of it with the large organizational goals. He is not responsible for enforcing any rules for the patient safety program.

31. A: This question indicates that employees feel disconnected from the administration of the organization and from the goals of the administration. In this situation, the healthcare quality management professional is responsible for helping create that connection – through a list of strategic goals, through a list of employee and administrative objectives, and through a mission statement. The healthcare quality management professional is unlikely to have the authority to organize committee meetings that review the changing policies, not in small part as this is more likely to increase the breach than to heal it.

32. B: Following the results of a risk management project, the healthcare quality management professional is responsible for helping the facility in applying the findings. Among the answer choices, the best option is for him to facilitate a performance improvement team that incorporates the findings into the larger organizational goals. Creating and disseminating a list of all employees is unlikely to accomplish much in the long term and certainly does little to ensure that the findings are integrated into the organization. Appointing an outside consultant may help, but it will not help as much as assembling an internal team that can then incorporate the findings into an organization it already knows well. Also, while developing a vision statement is helpful, it is a largely passive step and does little to create active improvement in risk management and prevention.

33. D: The facility is interested in finding out if the focus on customer satisfaction is effective. The best way to accomplish this is to provide patients and their families with surveys that allow them to respond. Contacting staff members might be helpful, but it does little to discover how much patients are directly affected by the facility's goals. Creating a performance improvement team with a focus on customer satisfaction is something that should already have occurred or that will occur, should the facility find out that its customer satisfaction goals have not yet been reached. And allowing employees to complain about negative experiences with patients and/or their families accomplishes little toward the goal of improving customer satisfaction.

34. C: The goal of educating facility staff members about patient safety should occur within the organization itself. Among the options for the process of education would include monthly email reminders, posted safety reminders, and occasional training events. Educating patients about facility goals for patient safety is unlikely to be a useful activity; what is more, patients already tend to be fairly focused on their own safety, and they are not necessarily responsible for the safety of other patients at the facility.

35. A: The healthcare quality management professional has the option of developing a plan for incorporating performance improvement findings into employee evaluations. He or she does not, however, have the authority to create a rewards hierarchy or generate an annual bonus plan for employees. Additionally, the option for sending out personalized messages to employees might be a

thoughtful gesture, but it hardly meets the facility's goal of quantifying the performance improvement team results.

36. C: The facility's goals of improved quality of care include several important areas – of increased safety, better nutrition, and staff friendliness. The healthcare quality management professional may certainly be involved in the following: developing an educational program that provides staff members with the tools to interact appropriately with patients, providing each department with friendly reminders about patient safety, and researching and providing the facility options to improve food quality. The healthcare quality management professional is unlikely, however, to be involved in creating a disciplinary process for unfriendly staff members.

37. A: In terms of licensing and/or accreditation, the healthcare quality management professional is responsible for communicating with the licensing/accrediting body and ensuring that any renewal is completed. The other answer choices contain shades of this idea but fail to express it as well as answer choice A. The healthcare quality management professional should certainly complete any necessary research on the licensing process, but he is unlikely to feel the need to locate a new licensing body simply because a renewal is imminent. He is likely to be part of the renewal process, but the task of completing the renewal documentation may or may not fall to this individual. He might also review staff activities to ensure compliance with the licensing requirements, but there may or may not be any need for the healthcare quality management professional to contact staff members directly about the renewal process.

38. D: Again, there is not necessarily a need to inform patients directly about the specific patient safety goals of the organization. The fact that the organization is committed to patient safety should be information enough. The healthcare quality management professional does have the responsibility to assist in the development of a patient safety culture within the organization, research technology options for improving the patient safety program, and incorporate patient safety goals within governance documents of the organization.

39. B: A degree of research would be appropriate in this situation, but the healthcare quality management professional is unlikely to include the research of contacting other hospitals. (The supporting research should come from official and/or scholarly sources.) The other answer choices reflect legitimate actions in this situation: evaluating the practice, reviewing the current standards, and comparing the policy to recommendations within the medical community.

40. C: Following the implementation of organizational change, the healthcare quality management professional's responsibility is to keep track of its effectiveness and to decide if there are any ongoing improvements to be made. As the change has already been implemented, there is no need to facilitate educational programs that begin the process of implementing it or to assemble performance improvement teams that continue integrating it. Surveying patients might be a useful step, but this depends entirely upon the type of change that has been implemented; in some cases, the change might be more internal, with patients knowing little about it and being unable to comment on it.

41. D: The best and most obvious way to prevent future instances of risk within the facility is to participate in revising the risk management plan to take the current findings into account. This is the role of the healthcare quality management professional, whose job is to be part of the overall management of quality healthcare within each facility. The other answer choices offer useful but incomplete options; i.e., identifying any employees who may have contributed to instances of risk, creating a new risk management program that utilizes technology, and educating employees about

how to avoid instances of risk. But each of these answer choices is too specific to provide the correct answer, which is broader in scope.

42. A: The healthcare quality management professional is authorized to develop a reward program that recognizes employees who contributed to patient safety. Answer choice B offers a valid option, but it does not answer the question as effectively as possible. The question indicates that the facility wants to reward successful employees, not discipline unsuccessful employees. Answer choices C and D also offer potentially correct actions for the healthcare quality management professional to take (with the exception of a ranking system, which does not necessarily fall under his or her job description); but again, neither really answers the question, which has to do with how to reward the specific employees who have contributed to the patient safety program.

43. D: The word "qualify" has a variety of meanings, one of which is "modify." The healthcare quality management professional certainly does not have the authority to modify data. He or she does, however, have the responsibility to define, collect, and summarize data.

44. B: One of the roles of the healthcare quality management professional is to evaluate accrediting bodies and assist the facility in selecting an appropriate accrediting body for voluntary accreditation. Answer choices A and C offer one part of this responsibility, but neither expresses it in full. Similarly, answer choice D offers an element of this responsibility but does not fully explain the role.

45. A: In terms of potential updates and improvements to a healthcare facility, the healthcare quality management professional should be part of the process of interpreting the data and supporting the decision-making process, in whatever form is expected, to apply updates and improvements. There is no need to appoint an advisor for this task; the healthcare quality management professional should be fully equipped for it already. The task of selecting updates is rather narrow and does not fall to the healthcare quality management professional alone. The task of applying the updates is certainly important, but once again it does not fall to the healthcare quality management professional alone; nor, it should be noted, is this the only role that he has in this process.

46. C: In the case of a regulatory body getting involved with a healthcare facility's activities, the healthcare quality management professional should take on the role of communicating with the regulatory body and ensuring a satisfactory solution to any problem(s). He should already be familiar with the standard rules and procedures of the regulatory body; this is not, however, the only part of his role. He is not necessarily in a position to be recommending disciplinary action, as it is likely that a standard for this is already in place. Finally, the regulatory body will provide the information about avoiding future errors, so the healthcare quality management professional does not need to do this as well.

47. B: Immediately following a performance improvement study, the primary role of the healthcare quality management professional is simple: begin applying the results of the study to the facility. Reviewing the results is important, but this does not necessarily create needed action. Disseminating information about the study is useful, but it depends entirely on the nature of the study and whether or not employees need to know about it directly. Evaluating the overall effectiveness of the study should be part of the follow-up task, but again the primary focus should be on applying the results.

48. D: The healthcare quality management professional is not responsible for recommending specific employees for promotion. (In some cases, this might be appropriate, but it is not necessarily part of his expectations.) The healthcare quality management professional, however, is responsible for assembling comparative data to measure employee performance, applying employee performance improvement to the facility evaluation system, and creating a program that recognizes employee performance improvement activities.

49. B: The term "mean" refers to the "average." It is unrelated to the probability, dispersion, or coefficient.

50. C: The standard deviation is the term that refers to any amount of variability from the mean, or average. The other terms – expected average, causality average, and observational error – have other meanings within statistical analysis.

51. C: It makes little sense for the healthcare quality management professional to create employee educational opportunities before the start of a performance improvement process. Education should follow the process, once the results have provided direction. Before starting the process, however, it is appropriate to develop outcome measurements for the performance improvement teams, assist in developing projects for them, and participate in establishing priorities for the performance improvement process.

52. D: In the case of a controversial practitioner decision, the role of the healthcare quality management professional is to evaluate the evidence from the practitioner's decision and compare the information to current practice guidelines. In other words, it is necessary to see if the decision is merited for future activities. The healthcare quality management professional should not need to contact a regulatory body except in the case of extreme variation from the practice guidelines (which is not indicated in the question). He might or might not interview staff members, but this would be part of the overall evaluation of the evidence. The decision to develop a performance improvement team would only be valid if it is determined that the practitioner's decision is inappropriate and calls for immediate changes. As this step would follow the immediate step of evaluation, the answer choice cannot be correct.

53. B: An unpredictable or fluctuating value is a random variation. Common and special cause variations reflect other types of variations that must be considered, but neither is described as unpredictable or fluctuating. A continuous variation is not a recognized term for statistical process control components.

54. C: The incident described in this question, that of a computer malfunction that alters otherwise expected activities, would be considered a special cause variation. In other words, the variation is due to a special cause that can be addressed and avoided in the future. This event does not describe a common or even random variation. A continuous variation is not a recognized term for statistical process control components.

55. C: In the event of a disparity in patient treatment due to unclear protocol, the role of the healthcare quality management professional is to participate in developing clinical guidelines for practitioners. Answer choices A and B reflect activities that might be part of the larger process of developing clinical guidelines. Answer choice D is not a priority; once the guidelines are in place and are followed, there should be no disparity in patient treatment. The clinic might choose to let patients know that changes have been made, but it is not necessarily the role of the healthcare quality management professional to make this decision or to present this information.

56. A: Question 55 reflects a common variation; that is, a variation that occurs commonly due to a lack of clear protocol. This is neither a random variation nor a special cause variation. Again, a continuous variation is not a recognized term for statistical process control components.

57. A: The healthcare quality management professional's role in employee evaluations is typically peripheral or subsidiary: that is to say, he should be part of the peripheral details involved with identifying and developing the benchmarks for job descriptions or the supporting activity of detailing employee activities. To create a ranking system for employees, however, does not necessarily fall under his job description. (For an educational comparison, the healthcare quality management professional is like the teaching assistant who grades the quizzes but does not make final decisions about each student's grade point average.) The healthcare quality management professional is qualified, however, to incorporate performance improvement findings into job appointment opportunities, to identify improved employee activities and apply these to the evaluation system that is already in place, and to recognize employees who have contributed to performance improvement through a privilege delineation system.

58. B: In this situation, the healthcare quality management professional should create a budget and complete cost-analysis reviews to ensure that the performance improvement plan does not exceed the allotted amount. As a healthcare quality management professional is not a marketing executive, he is not responsible for creating fundraising opportunities for the clinic. Additionally, it would not be appropriate in this situation for him to attempt to cut costs elsewhere to allow for performance improvement spending; the correct task in this case is simply to stay on budget. Answer choice D contains elements of the correct answer, but it is vague about "opportunities to reduce costs" – with no indication of where these costs will be cut. The correct answer is the more direct one: create a budget, and stick to it by keeping a close eye on cost and spending.

59. A: The decision to maintain the confidentiality of performance improvement results depends entirely on the nature of the performance improvement activity. In some cases, it might not be necessary to broadcast the results; in most cases, it would be acceptable and even appropriate. The healthcare quality management professional should, however, maintain the confidentiality of activities, reports, and records during the completion of the performance improvement process.

60. C: For a new data collection system, the healthcare quality management professional should be part of the task of developing a methodology for data collection. In other words, he should assist the facility in creating a clear method suited to the type of data and how it needs to be collected. The process of developing a data collection methodology might involve informing the facility about regulatory requirements, but this would simply be one part of the larger process. Similarly, creating a confidentiality program for the data and researching data collection systems might be part of the larger process of defining the data collection methodology, instead of the only part.

61. A: Follow-up activities for a revamped patient safety program do not necessarily include informing patients of their rights as accorded by state and federal law. Patients should certainly be made aware of these rights, but this particular activity is largely irrelevant to the situation described in question 61. The healthcare quality management professional does have the responsibility of educating employees about the patient safety program goals, reviewing these goals periodically to see if they are being assimilated into the organization, and developing opportunities to integrate these goals into the organization.

62. C: The healthcare quality management professional's job entails participation in a medical record review, peer review, and service specific review. It does not typically involve participation in a review of the facility's governance, which is determined by a higher authority.

63. A: Utilizing technology for a patient safety program typically involves researching available software and assisting in selecting the best software option for the facility. Working with the IT department might be part of this process, but it is only one part and too narrow to describe the full responsibility of the healthcare quality management professional in the situation. Sending out email reminders and providing patient safety information on the facility's website, again, might be part of the process, but both fail to embrace the full scope of applying technology for a patient safety program.

64. B: The healthcare quality management professional is responsible for integrating performance improvements into the facility's by-laws, administrative policies, and procedures. It is unlikely that he will apply them to committee meetings, particularly since these meetings are likely part of the performance improvement process itself.

65. D: Following an audit, the healthcare quality management professional should take steps to integrate the results of the audit into the facility's goals and activities. Answer choices A, B, and C reflect individual steps in this larger goal, but each is too narrow to be the best option.

66. C: The performance improvement results will be available after the performance improvement process has begun. So it makes no sense to review the results as a part of getting started on the performance improvement process: there are not yet any results to review. The healthcare quality management professional can, however, establish strategic goals, develop performance improvement activities, and create projects for the performance improvement teams.

67. A: The Malcolm Baldridge Award recognizes organizational excellence in a facility, and it is also presented by the President. The other answer choices represent healthcare awards offered for different occasions; additionally, none is presented by the President.

68. C: The Magnet Designation specifically recognizes excellence in nursing. The other answer choices represent healthcare awards offered for different occasions; additionally, focuses on nursing as the Magnet Designation does.

69. A: The healthcare quality management professional's role is to review the standards for the award and determine the feasibility in applying for it. The other answer choices indicate elements of this correct answer; namely, developing performance improvement projects to address any problems, contacting the awards committee to understand the application process, and comparing benchmarking data from other facilities Only answer choice A, however, summarizes all of this into a single statement.

70. B: In this situation, as in others, the role of the healthcare quality management professional is somewhat peripheral. That is to say, he should simply take part in reviewing the evidence about the decision and in offering the facility information to assist with making the best ongoing decision. This role of assistance may or may not include a performance improvement team; it would first be necessary to review the situation as a whole. Additionally, the role of assisting the facility may or may not entail asking the fast food chain to remove unhealthy options or locating other fast food chains to increase customer options. But again, the first and primary step is to take a careful look at everything and provide the facility with the information it needs to make decisions.

71. C: In the case of an internal supply dispute, the primary role of the healthcare quality management professional is to assist the facility in clarifying the supply relationship between departments and in reviewing the process for ordering supplies. The other answer choices represent steps in part of this process (appointing a new supply manager, researching the error in communication breakdown, assessing and recommending a software program), but individually none of them encompasses the fullness of the healthcare quality management professional's role.

72. D: Answer choice D provides the complete answer for the role of the healthcare quality management professional in the case of an external supplier; he takes on the responsibility of supporting the facility first and foremost, as well as of assisting the facility in establishing the best contractual relationship with the supplier. This role might (or might not) include the other answer choice options – researching different supplier firms, considering the ratings of the supplier firms, and drawing up the contract itself. The primary role, however, is one of support for the facility.

73. B: In the case of assessing and improving the quality culture, the healthcare quality management professional should review the organization's activities and develop a performance improvement program to apply necessary changes. Once again, the other answer choices provide elements of this, but they are too specific to encompass the full role of the healthcare quality management professional.

74. D: A Pareto chart is, with its combination of a bar graph and a line graph, most useful for determining the most important factor among a large group of factors. A control chart is useful for seeing the changes in a process. A fishbone chart is most useful for helping to determine cause and effect. A run chart is most useful for viewing data over a time sequence.

75. C: A run chart is most useful for viewing data over a time sequence. A control chart is useful for seeing the changes in a process. A fishbone chart is most useful for helping to determine cause and effect. A Pareto chart is most useful for determining the most important factor among a large group of factors.

76. A: A control chart is most useful for seeing the changes in a process, and thus for determining whether or not a process is stable. A fishbone chart is most useful for helping to determine cause and effect. A run chart is most useful for viewing data over a time sequence. A Pareto chart is most useful for determining the most important factor among a large group of factors.

77. D: Linking the performance improvement of a facility to its strategic goals is unlikely to include informing patients of their legal rights within that facility – unless patient rights are part of the specific performance improvement process. As the question does not indicate, it is impossible to assume this as an immediate option for ways the healthcare quality management professional can connect performance improvement to strategic goals. The other answer choices (identifying clear strategic goals, developing performance improvement activities, and educating staff members) all represent direct ways to create this link.

78. C: CPOE stands for Computerized Physician Order Entry and is thus an electronic entry process for physicians or practitioners to create patient treatment instructions. EMR stands for Electronic Medical Record; BCMA stands for Bar Code Medication Administration; JCI stands for Joint Commission International.

79. B: BCMA, which stands for Bar Code Medication Administration, was designed for doctors and nurses to ensure that they are treating the correct patient with the correct medicine, at the correct

dose, and to avoid any medical errors. CPOE stands for Computerized Physician Order Entry. JCI stands for Joint Commission International.

80. A: EMR stands for Electronic Medical Record and is a type of computerized patient record that is maintained within a local healthcare facility. It is typically not linked to other patient record systems. BCMA stands for Bar Code Medication Administration. CPOE stands for Computerized Physician Order Entry. JCI stands for Joint Commission International.

81. A: The role of the healthcare quality management professional in this situation is to interpret the incident report and assist the facility's administration in applying procedures to avoid future errors. Beyond this, the healthcare quality management professional relies on the guidance of the facility. He may or may not be asked to note the incident in the practitioner's profile, but this will be determined by the facility administration. The creation of a performance improvement project would result from a review of the incident report and the recommendation of the administration. The healthcare quality management professional might decide to advise a suspension of the practitioner, but again this would result from a review of the report.

82. D: In terms of benchmarking data, the healthcare quality management professional should review the facility's performance and compare it to other facilities in the same class (e.g., clinics, hospitals). Research is likely to be involved, but the application of industry standards will come from a knowledge of these standards or further research in looking into them. A marketing campaign is the responsibility of the facility's marketing professional and not of the healthcare quality management professional. The facilitation of performance improvement projects would occur after the review of the facility and a comparison to benchmarking data.

83. B: To prepare for upcoming licensure, the healthcare quality management professional should be involved in reviewing licensure expectations, preparing appropriate survey training, and developing and facilitating educational opportunities for staff members. The evaluation of performance improvement activities should follow directly after the completion of those activities and is not (necessarily) related directly to preparing for licensure. As a result, answer choice B indicates a potentially irrelevant step and cannot be correct.

84. C: The situation posed in question 84 would require a t-test, which is typically used to determine the difference in averages between two samples. For instance, the t-test would be useful for seeing how the average of the medication group compares to the average of the placebo group. Regression analysis is used to consider a dependent variable against a number of other independent variables. Probability analysis and parametric analysis are not recognized types of testing analyses.

85. A: Regression analysis is used to consider a dependent variable against a number of other independent variables. In this case, the dependent variable is the health regime, and the independent variables are the various backgrounds and lifestyles of the patients. A t-test is used to determine the difference in averages between two samples. Probability analysis and parametric analysis are not recognized types of testing analyses.

86. A: The question asks for the first step that should occur before assembling a performance improvement team. The only answer that can be correct in this case is the answer that reflects a collection of information, i.e., answer choice A. The identification of patient safety goals is only relevant if patient safety goals are part of the performance improvement project. With no information to indicate this, answer choice B is largely irrelevant. Communicating with an

accreditation body makes little sense in this situation. Surveying customers would, like answer choice B, only be relevant if the performance improvement project required direct customer input. With no information to indicate this, the best answer can only be option A.

87. C: The healthcare quality management professional contributes to the development of survey processes for accreditation, safety policy, and licensure. He does not necessarily get involved with survey processes for governance, unless specifically required to do so.

88. D: Direct practitioner management is more likely to fall under the domain of the administrative board. The healthcare quality management professional, however, can expect to get involved with care management, disease management, and case management (all of which fall under the more general heading of "utilization management").

89. B: The balanced scorecard represents a way to connect the activities of an organization to its larger strategies. The dashboard represents a collection of all performance data from within an organization. The term core measures is derived from a national performance system developed by Joint Commission. Quality management is a more general term that refers to the consideration, direction, and overall management of quality goals within a facility.

90. A: The dashboard represents a collection of all performance data from within an organization. The balanced scorecard represents a way to connect the activities of an organization to its larger strategies. The term core measures is derived from a national performance system developed by Joint Commission. Quality management is a more general term that refers to the consideration, direction, and overall management of quality goals within a facility.

91. D: The term core measures is derived from a national performance system developed by Joint Commission. The dashboard represents a collection of all performance data from within an organization. The balanced scorecard represents a way to connect the activities of an organization to its larger strategies. Quality management is a more general term that refers to the consideration, direction, and overall management of quality goals within a facility.

92. C: Sometimes the simplest and most obvious answer is also the correct one. The primary role of the healthcare quality management professional for the integration of quality concepts is in defining the quality concepts for the organization and developing ways to incorporate these concepts into day-to-day activities. The creation of training programs, the review of benchmarking data, and the incorporation of quality concepts into the employee appraisal system all fall under this larger category, but all are too specific to encompass the full role.

93. A: The healthcare quality management professional can expect to collect, define, and summarize data. He may need to delegate these tasks, but to "delegate data" makes little sense and cannot be the correct answer choice.

94. B: Research has shown that the biggest effect on the failure of an organization to correctly apply medical ethics to patients is related to the breakdown of communication within the facility. A failed application of medical ethics is far less likely to be connected to poorly trained staff members (because patient treatment is a priority in staff training), unclear information about legal requirements or inconsistency between state and federal expectations (because the ethics themselves may or may not have legal support or state/federal mandates).

95. C: In terms of risk management, the healthcare quality management professional can expect to collaborate with the quality department, analyze failures in risk management, and coordinate risk management activities. The review of medical records has no immediate connection to risk management, and without further indication to create a connection answer choice C must be correct.

96. A: To link risk management to performance improvement, the healthcare quality management professional should expect to complete a risk management assessment—that is, review the facility's current risk management process(es) —and then integrate this assessment into the performance improvement activities. Answer choice B approaches a correct answer but does not encompass the idea clearly; yes, the healthcare quality management professional should detail risk prevention activities, but identifying opportunities for updating or redefining performance improvement goals is a fairly passive activity that does not clearly suggest integration. Similarly, answer choice C contains elements of the correct answer, but it fails by focusing only on the major causes of risk. A solid risk management approach looks at all forms of risk. While the assembly of a performance improvement team is useful, it is not necessarily the only approach to performance improvement, nor is it the only way to connect performance improvement and risk management.

97. D: For the healthcare quality management professional, risk management as applied to a patient safety program has three focuses: the analysis of the root cause of a failure, the review of an incident report detailing the failure, and the evaluation of the event that triggered the failure. The application of patient advocacy laws is a different area altogether and has only a peripheral connection to risk management and a patient safety program.

98. B: In this scenario, the healthcare quality management professional should facilitate ongoing communication between the department and the administration, as well as participate in a review of the current procedures. There is an inherent goal of establishing clear lines of authority, but the department might be making a good point about unnecessary steps in the procedure. At the same time, procedure exists for a reason, so communication and discussion must occur to arrive at an appropriate solution. The facilitation of communication and the review of the procedure might involve a review committee, but the review committee by itself is not the only responsibility of the healthcare quality management professional. Answer choice C is an option that would result from a careful review of the situation and the procedure, but it is certainly not the action to take before a review occurs. Answer choice D contains a piece of the correct answer—that is, a review—but the facilitation of communication is also a necessary part, due to the potential breakdown of authority lines in this situation.

99. D: Question 99 presents a perfect example of the need for performance improvement. It is likely that mistakes have occurred on both sides—the supervisor's and the employees'. As a result, the healthcare quality management professional can apply performance improvement activities to the situation with two major goals in mind: the education of both supervisor and employees regarding their respective roles and the establishment of an effective working relationship between the two groups in the department. Answer choice A contains part of the correct answer: mediation should occur. But it is not the only thing that should occur, and therefore the option is not correct. Answer choice B also contains potentially good information; it is important to maintain the lines of authority in the facility, thus the employees should be reminded about the supervisor's role. There is also, however, a very good chance that the supervisor needs a reminder about respecting employees, therefore the action taken in answer choice B is not sufficient. Answer choice C accomplishes little. To move the supervisor simply relocates the potential for a problem to another department. Without further information about what caused the breakdown in authority, it makes

- 41 -

no sense to sweep it under the rug by moving a person who might very well need leadership training. There is always the chance that the same problems will arise in the new department; therefore, answer choice C is a passive approach with no effort made to improve the situation.

100. C: A statement about intended profits belongs in board rooms and committee meetings. Even for a publicly traded company, the discussion of profits does not belong in a vision statement. This reduces the vision statement to a purely venal goal and strips it of appeal. The vision statement should, however, discuss the expected outcomes (non-monetary), the operational goals, and the personalized approach to an image. The last, it should be noted, gives the vision statement a unique shape and avoids too generic a presentation of the organization.

101. A: Once again, the simplest and most obvious answer is correct. A department needs a new supplier for major elements of its inventory. The healthcare quality management professional can help by researching, identifying, and recommending a new supplier. The documentation to end the relationship with the old supplier has likely been completed already, particularly since the question notes that the department "has ended" the relationship. Creating a list of potential suppliers is helpful, but the healthcare quality management professional's role can exceed this. In the same way, evaluating the available suppliers and reviewing their contract expectations is part of the role, but is not the only part of the role.

102. A: Question 102 reflects a common variation: that of bad equipment maintenance that creates common, albeit unnecessary, failures. In other words, a common variation is a variation that occurs commonly due to a lack of clear protocol or procedure. A random variation is unpredictable (and poorly maintained equipment can be predicted to fail). A special cause variation is also unpredictable, but it is more the result of unexpected events that have no recognizable history of having occurred, rather than pure randomness. A continuous variation is not a recognized term for a statistical variation.

103. A: This scenario is also a common variation. The working conditions affect the outcome, and consistently poor working conditions can be a recognized part of a variable outcome in patient care. A random variation is unpredictable. A special cause variation is also unpredictable, but it is more the result of unexpected events that have no recognizable history of having occurred, rather than pure randomness. A continuous variation is not a recognized term for a statistical variation.

104. C: A doctor's failure to adjust the patient settings can be viewed as a special cause variation. The fault is not that of the equipment, but rather that of the doctor who did not use the equipment correctly. For the healthcare facility, it might be difficult to anticipate such an event without having encountered it first. A common variation is a variation that occurs commonly due to a lack of clear protocol or procedure. (After this experience, it might be that the facility applies a protocol for this type of treatment; a doctor who fails to follow it after that will reflect a common variation instead of a special cause variation.) A random variation is unpredictable. A continuous variation is not a recognized term for a statistical variation.

105. B: A tornado that veers off its expected course is a random variation. A common variation is a variation that occurs commonly due to a lack of clear protocol or procedure. A special cause variation is also unpredictable, but it is more the result of unexpected events that have no recognizable history of having occurred, rather than pure randomness. (Tornados have certainly occurred before; in this scenario, the tornado was largely random because it was not expected to move in the direction it did.) A continuous variation is not a recognized term for a statistical variation.

106. C: The patients' mood during treatment is not really quantifiable, so this would be considered qualitative data. The other options—blood pressure readings, changes in weight, and cholesterol levels—are quantifiable and are thus considered quantitative data.

107. B: The behavior of employees to customers is qualitative; that is to say, it's more a measure of quality than of quantity. The other options—paper records maintained by the department, average hours worked by each employee, and productivity rate of the department—can be quantified, so these represent quantifiable data.

108. B: In this situation, the role of the healthcare quality management professional is to assist a healthcare facility in determining who is responsible for what in the facility, while also working with departments to ensure a clear flow of communication. As a result, answer choice B best reflects his responsibility; that is, to mediate between the departments and help to ensure a clear understanding of roles. Additionally, the healthcare quality management professional should also follow up with patients about treatment, establishing a flow of communication between the patients and the facility. In other words, answer choice B summarizes the full role of the healthcare quality management professional. Answer choice A, however, reflects only part of the role; that is, to present to each department the information about its current responsibilities. Unless there is indication that one (or both) of the departments has deliberately failed in its activities or has failed due to serious procedural problems, no citation would be necessary. What is more, this would not necessarily be the task of the healthcare quality management professional. Communication with the patients might be appropriate, but it is certainly not the only responsibility of the healthcare quality management professional in this situation.

109. A: The primary role of the healthcare quality management professional in this situation would be to assist the department in setting up a manageable budget and working within it. Answer choices B, C, and D indicate parts of this process (communicating between the department and the facility, establishing a clear budget for the department, and reviewing the department's activities for ways to cut costs), but none of them summarizes the full responsibility of the healthcare quality management professional.

110. A: It is not necessarily the responsibility of the healthcare quality management professional to make cuts in staff salaries. What is more, it is unlikely that a healthcare facility would dip into staff salaries to find money for a program. The healthcare quality management professional is, however, responsible for supporting the facility in setting up a budget, providing a cost analysis to ensure a good cost-return ratio, and researching potentially unexpected costs.

111. C: Utilizing historical data is not necessarily an essential part of performance improvement measurement. (In fact, historical data can actually be a negative as a performance improvement measurement when it prevents a facility from making progress by trusting past results.) Evaluating the productivity of employee activities, reviewing the effectiveness of technology, and comparing the facility's performance to that of other facilities all represent useful performance improvement measurements.

112. D: In this situation, the healthcare quality management professional should assist the hospital in responding to customer complaints and in reviewing options for integrating a new policy. It may turn out that a new policy is not feasible, but if enough complaints arise the facility might very well take a close look at the policy. The healthcare quality management professional might review the policy, but he will only encourage the facility to make changes if the changes are feasible. In other words, no change is guaranteed. A communication process for customers would be appropriate, but

- 43 -

it is not the healthcare quality management professional's only responsibility in this case. The healthcare quality management professional would submit to family members a copy of (and explanation for) the policy if there is no decision to change the policy.

113. A: Answer choice A summarizes the entire responsibility of the healthcare quality management professional in this case. Answer choices B, C, and D reflect elements of this role – reviewing the systems to select the most effective one, considering the details of all available systems to ensure they meet the standards, and submitting a recommendation for a system – but none of these options encompasses the full responsibility.

114. A: A scattergram chart is most useful for comparing two different variables of data. A line graph is useful for considering the change in data over time. A bar graph is useful for indicating the probability of change in data. A pie chart is useful for specifying the proportion of each variable.

115. B: A performance improvement plan does not necessarily need to include comparative research of external performance improvement plans. A performance improvement plan should, however, include a defined list of priorities among the performance improvement activities, a clear definition of the performance improvement problem that needs to be addressed, and an established list of standards to be met during performance improvement.

116. D: Among the answer choices, the best option is D: organizational transparency in a healthcare facility means active leadership to ensure the public image matches the private image as closely as possible. In other words, there should be little difference between what happens behind the scenes and what is presented to the public. Complete public availability of records might be important for some corporations, but it is not necessarily the best definition of organizational transparency for a healthcare facility. A full presentation of goals, objectives, and standards on a website is part of organizational transparency, but it is only one part. Similarly, public accountability for mistakes that occur is a part, but it is not the only part of organizational transparency for healthcare facility.

117. C: Organizational transparency does not necessarily include a public explanation of all activities within the facility. That could rapidly prove to be a logistical—as well as a public relations—nightmare. Organizational transparency tends to be more standard: an annual report about facility costs and activities, a public statement about facility values, and clear information about facility partnerships (i.e., who has a stake in activities, and who does not; whether there is any potential for a conflict of interests).

118. D: The by-laws within a healthcare facility are simply the list of organizational "laws" that define activities and procedures within the facility. In other words, by-laws are internal expectations. They are not state and federal guidelines (although they might reflect state and federal laws), legal conditions for patient treatment and practitioner activity, or a list of patient rights and ethics.

119. A: Utilization management is essentially an assessment of different healthcare services based on whether those services are necessary and efficient. Answer choices B, C, and D—an internal review of facility procedures based on federal standards, a self-review of facility activities by a licensed group of experienced professionals, and a measurement of facility performance to accommodate internal and external standards—do not reflect utilization management. It should be noted, however, that answer choice C reflects a peer review, while answer choice D reflects performance measurement.

120. C: A peer review is not part of utilization management. Case management, demand management, and disease management are, however, part of utilization management. (The fourth part of utilization management is care management.)

121. A: In this situation, the healthcare quality management professional is responsible for monitoring all consultant activity to ensure that it meets standards for quality and patient safety. Answer choices B, C, and D reflect potential elements of this responsibility (researching the history of consultant activity, communicating expectations to consultants, and assembling a review team to ensure consultants fulfill expectations), but none of these options encompass the role in full.

122. D: A self-directed team is best for a project that requires a measure of autonomy and can complete tasks with limited oversight. A cross-functional team is best for combining employees with different skill sets and areas of experience to complete a task. A work group is a more general term for a group of individuals who work together on a project. A quality circle is typically composed of volunteers who assist with problem solving.

123. A: A cross-functional team is best for combining employees with different skill sets and areas of experience to complete a task. A work group is a more general term for a group of individuals who work together on a project. A quality circle is typically composed of volunteers who assist with problem solving. A self-directed team is best for a project that requires a measure of autonomy and can complete tasks with limited oversight.

124. B: While a clear leader might seem like an obvious part of a team, a leader is not necessarily part of every team. (For instance, a self-directed team has no leader, as the name suggests. All team members simply work together toward a common goal.) A team should, however, have a solid sense of its goals and responsibilities, good internal relationships among team members, and a willingness to discuss the effectiveness of decisions and activities.

125. A: Previous experience in working on a team might be useful, but it is not necessarily an essential part of considering people for a new team. In fact, someone with no previous team experience might very well prove to be a great asset if he has the other qualities listed: personal strengths and skill set(s), effective problem-solving abilities, and an ability to listen and contribute.

Practice Test #2

Practice Questions

1. Which of the following is the best definition of "vision" in regards to creating an organizational vision statement?
   a. The ability to see the future
   b. An ideal future state
   c. A realistic action plan for future performance
   d. An outline of future organizational purpose

2. A patient care team is in disagreement over new admissions procedures. What decision-making model should management use?
   a. Decision criteria
   b. Consensus
   c. Invocation
   d. Tenure influence

3. St. Joseph's Hospital was recently ranked last in the region in the area of efficiency in transferring patients to inpatient beds. When working on process improvements, what type of data is likely to prove most helpful?
   a. Internal data
   b. Historical data
   c. Quality control data
   d. Comparative data

4. Which of the following is a structure designed to help facilitate team or group pursuit of specific goals and objectives?
   a. Management
   b. Organization
   c. Intelligent design
   d. Delegation

5. Mrs. Jones waits more than an hour past her scheduled appointment time. She finally leaves in a huff, calling the doctor's office a joke and saying she has better things to do. Mrs. Jones' perception of quality in this instance is based on...
   a. Medical care.
   b. Statistical anomalies.
   c. Provider norms.
   d. Patient care.

6. If managers fail to make organizational decisions consciously, what generally serves as the basis for outcomes?
   a. Circumstances
   b. Organizational policy
   c. Statistical norms
   d. Federal regulations

7. During a surgical procedure, a small medical implement was left inside a patient. The follow-up surgery to remove the implement is an example of...
 a. Quality improvement.
 b. Quality control.
 c. Quality assurance.
 d. Total quality.

8. Which of the following statements about quality in healthcare is true?
 a. Quality is a conglomerate of lessons, methods, and knowledge.
 b. Quality directly correlates to patient safety.
 c. Quality is multifaceted and multidimensional in nature.
 d. All of the above

9. Which of the following is not considered a principle of total quality?
 a. Competent management
 b. Customer focus
 c. Continuous improvement
 d. Teamwork

10. Healthcare organizations are often classified as systems. What is the primary reason for this designation?
 a. They span several states with a network of providers.
 b. They are dynamically complex and have multiple levels of management.
 c. They are a collection of parts that function as an interdependent whole.
 d. They employ a broad cross-section of the population in various positions.

11. Mary has a family history of heart disease and type II diabetes. She also has pre-hypertension. Mary's doctor recently put her on a diet and exercise program. This is an example of system thinking called...
 a. Quality control.
 b. Preemptive medicine.
 c. Continuous improvement.
 d. History dependency.

12. How does the World Health Organization Surgical Safety Checklist lead to tight coupling in the operating room?
 a. It establishes universality for patients.
 b. It compartmentalizes the procedures.
 c. It establishes a clear operating room hierarchy.
 d. It closely aligns the various individuals involved in the process.

13. Who created the hospital information management standard that states, "The hospital maintains the security and integrity of health information?"
 a. The Baldrige Committee
 b. The Joint Commission
 c. The National Institutes of Health
 d. The ORYX Initiative

14. The rate of sick days among employees in the intensive care unit (ICU) falls well within the hospital standard, but the CNAs claim the RNs take too many sick days, and this prevents consistent

care relationships between RNs and CNAs. What should management do to investigate this situation?

    a. Set up surveillance of the department
    b. Distribute patient surveys throughout the ICU
    c. Distribute employee surveys throughout the ICU
    d. Unbundle/disaggregate the data and reanalyze it

15. The new administrator of Hospital A implements a top-down hand washing policy for all employees and visitors to the hospital. As a result, previously high infection rates drop below national standard levels for the first time. This new policy is an example of...

    a. Performance measures.
    b. Quality assurance.
    c. Risk management.
    d. Information management.

16. The Baldrige Performance Excellence Program Health Care Criteria remark on the importance of measurement and analysis of data. What can be the downside of a heavy performance data focus?

    a. Managers can get tunnel vision and overlook non-measured errors and issues.
    b. Data far above the national standard can result in inflated self-opinion.
    c. Data far below the national standard can result in depression and despondency.
    d. Hospitals with high data scores are held to impossibly high standards.

17. A position has recently opened for a department head in human resources (HR). It is your job to select the best internal candidate to interview for the position. Which of the following candidates possesses the strongest leadership potential?

    a. An HR supervisor who has been with the organization for 10 years.
    b. An accounting supervisor who has a perfect quality record.
    c. An HR employee who mentors new hires and frequently attends voluntary training.
    d. A supervisor in the maintenance department who wants to try something new.

18. In a large hospital setting, which of the following represents an internal customer?

    a. An admitted patient
    b. A physical therapy department assistant
    c. A medical equipment supplier
    d. A patient's family

19. Who should be considered when developing process requirements within a healthcare organization?

    a. Patients
    b. Internal customers
    c. Stakeholders
    d. All of the above

20. What happens right after a Joint Commission-accredited hospital experiences a sentinel event?

    a. An award is presented to administrators.
    b. A root cause analysis is performed.
    c. Immediate re-accreditation is granted.
    d. Performance improvement measures are implemented.

21. A small city has two hospitals. The Hospital Consumer Assessment of Healthcare Providers and Systems (HCAHPS) reports show Hospital A is performing far below Hospital B in customer service. The administrators at Hospital A decide to set an organizational goal of ranking higher than Hospital B in customer service in one year. What is the most logical first step in the goal-setting process?
    a. Develop an overall picture of the partial goals to be achieved.
    b. Identify a specific and singular goal to be initially pursued.
    c. Require immediate training for all members of each department.
    d. Bring in customer service experts to evaluate and improve processes.

22. The process improvement team has recently established a goal that all patients be triaged within 20 minutes of arrival in the emergency room (ER). What might be a negative outcome of this goal?
    a. ER nurses will be overstressed.
    b. Mistakes are likely to be made.
    c. Triage will be less thorough.
    d. All of the above

23. Which of the following can be defined as, "A set of measures and data that give managers and administrators a quick yet comprehensive overview of performance?"
    a. Process measurement
    b. Balanced scorecard
    c. Dashboard
    d. Six Sigma

24. Within the last four days, three post-surgical patients have died of pneumonia complications at a large hospital. None of the patients presented as symptomatic for pneumonia at the time of surgery. What evaluation tool should be used to help identify and resolve this issue?
    a. Epidemiological theory
    b. Performance management measures
    c. Statistical analysis
    d. Improvement measures

25. What is the primary purpose of the Consumer Assessment of Health Providers and Systems (CAHPS)?
    a. To relieve data collection efforts by administrators
    b. To offer patients an anonymous outlet for healthcare complaints
    c. To capture patient satisfaction data in a universal manner
    d. To provide a forum for more effective communication between patients and providers

26. When Hospital A's neonatal infection rates rise unexpectedly, the quality council establishes a new set of performance measures. They base their measures on internal standards, customer survey data, and employee survey data. What important element are the quality council members disregarding?
    a. Epidemiological standards
    b. Customer satisfaction data
    c. Employment records
    d. External standards

27. What challenge often occurs with the use of aggregated data?
    a. The numbers become too large to comprehend.
    b. Context is lost and solutions are not identified.
    c. Impersonality and vagueness are not engaging.
    d. Special interpreters are needed for understanding.

28. As a quality professional, you are about to address administrators regarding a recent decrease in customer satisfaction with postpartum care. In preparation, you want to create a report to present at the meeting. Which of the following would be most important to consider as you prepare your report?
    a. Properly formatting the report to industry standards
    b. Identifying the data most relevant to the situation
    c. Expounding on historical data on postpartum care
    d. Reviewing postpartum satisfaction at other organizations

29. Which of the following is a good way to assess customer needs and expectations?
    a. Surveys
    b. Focus groups
    c. Informal discussions
    d. All of the above

30. Which of the following is the most important way that transparency of healthcare data serves as a regulator for the industry?
    a. It encourages performance improvement to create more positive data.
    b. It tends to drive poorly-performing organizations out of business.
    c. It creates a culture of shame and fear among employees.
    d. It does not serve any regulatory purpose.

31. Which of the following is the logical first priority in process improvement?
    a. Training employees on improvements
    b. Measuring process improvement
    c. Identifying process issues
    d. Creating an improvement plan

32. As a manager, you are working with a new employee who has challenges with appropriate customer service processes. Together you are establishing a performance improvement plan. Which of the following should not be a part of the plan?
    a. Research into the causes of the employee's challenges
    b. A clear statement of the problems to be addressed
    c. Specific action steps to be taken as part of the plan
    d. A desired outcome or goal behavior and a timeline

33. What role do clinical guidelines play in establishing process requirements for an organization?
    a. They conflict with one another.
    b. Clinical guidelines dictate process requirements.
    c. Process requirements dictate clinical guidelines.
    d. They are unrelated.

34. Recent HCAHPS data for Hospital A indicate that doctors are not providing adequate explanations to patients. In improving the patient safety culture with regards to this issue, what two elements must be addressed?
   a. Patient perceptions and clinical quality
   b. Patient perceptions and physician education
   c. Physician education and time constraints
   d. Quality standards and time constraints

35. Which of the following is a patient safety goal identified by the Joint Commission?
   a. Cut service times in emergency departments
   b. Apply Six Sigma principles to sentinel events
   c. Improve the effectiveness of caregiver communications
   d. Establish strong customer service numbers among patients

36. How might an implicit organizational goal of service time reduction be an accidental adversary to patient safety goals?
   a. They could not be accidental adversaries.
   b. A rush to meet service times might impede adequate communication.
   c. Improved service times may negatively impact service levels.
   d. Customer satisfaction levels might be falsely elevated.

37. In a quest to improve patient satisfaction data, Clinic A is creating a patient survey. Which of the following areas should be the focus of the survey?
   a. Physical needs
   b. Emotional needs
   c. Social needs
   d. All of the above

38. At a business lunch, a colleague from a hospital across town encourages you to try implementing Six Sigma to improve your organization. After discussing it at length with your colleague, you feel the biggest benefit of Six Sigma for your hospital would be,
   a. The goal of driving errors to zero.
   b. The long-standing tradition of use.
   c. The origins in manufacturing.
   d. The view that all work is a process.

39. Two hospitals in your region have recently adopted computerized physician order entry (CPOE). You have assembled an evaluation team to determine if CPOE is right for your organization. Which of the following factors would likely have the strongest impact on your decision?
   a. It is important for your organization to be technologically competitive.
   b. Several patients and healthcare providers have endorsed the system.
   c. The system is shown to reduce prescribing errors by 50 percent or more.
   d. Major stakeholders are pressuring for adoption of the system.

40. The intensive care unit (ICU) is facing a problem with excessive sick days being taken by the CNA staff. After surveying ICU employees, you identify several potential causes for this issue. When you present this information to the management team, what type of visual representation would be most effective?
    a. A flowchart or deployment chart
    b. A pie chart or run chart
    c. A fishbone diagram or Pareto chart
    d. None of the above

41. What type of data analysis is most appropriate after an organization experiences a significant negative event?
    a. Prospective analysis
    b. Root cause analysis
    c. Failure mode and effects analysis
    d. Introspective analysis

42. An issue with response time to patient requests has been identified in the post-surgical ward of Hospital A. The administrators desire to improve performance in this area. What element of process performance will most help determine the best course of action?
    a. Process behavior
    b. Process measurement
    c. Process capability
    d. Process requirements

43. In what way are benchmark data valuable to the performance improvement process?
    a. They provide a comparison standard for behavior.
    b. They can be used to punish underperformers.
    c. They can be used to reward high performers.
    d. They assist in achieving department-specific accreditation.

44. Which of the following is absolutely essential for the leader of an effective performance improvement team?
    a. "Type A" personality
    b. Charisma and persuasion
    c. Modeling target behaviors
    d. Extended tenure with the organization

45. Who developed the National Patient Safety Goals (NPSGs)?
    a. The Leapfrog Group
    b. HCAHPS
    c. Centers for Disease Control (CDC)
    d. The Joint Commission

46. Over the past year, Hospital A has become much busier, and there have been several significant medication administration errors. Management is determined to rectify this issue as quickly and efficiently as possible. Which of the following would be the best solution for patient safety?
    a. Retraining nursing staff on medication administration
    b. Implementing barcode medication administration technology
    c. Shortening nursing shifts to increase alertness
    d. Requiring two-person teams to administrate medications

47. Hospital B implemented a performance improvement and total quality overhaul just over a year ago. Upon analysis of financial data for this year, Hospital B discovers increased profits in spite of training costs for the program. What is the most likely reason for this profitability?
    a. There was an accounting error.
    b. All hospitals in the area saw profits.
    c. Increased quality drew new customers.
    d. Most of the staff took a pay cut.

48. As a department manager, you notice increasing absences and decreasing performance levels among CNAs in your department. What could you do to help identify the cause of these issues?
    a. Distribute employee satisfaction surveys
    b. Organize employee feedback forums
    c. Aggregate and carefully evaluate relevant statistical data
    d. All of the above

49. How does use of an electronic medical record (EMR) improve patient safety?
    a. Any use of technology reduces errors in healthcare.
    b. EMR brings an organization up to national standards.
    c. EMR provides all patient information in a centralized place.
    d. Using EMR does not improve patient safety.

50. As a manager, you see a need to strengthen patient safety within your organization. What is the most effective way to introduce new patient safety measures into your organizational culture?
    a. Integrate patient safety measures into existing strategic goals
    b. Provide extensive mandatory training on patient safety
    c. Assemble managers and require them to roll policies down to employees
    d. Create a new set of organizational goals solely based on patient safety

51. As manager of information technology, you feel your responsibility for risk management is minimal. What risk management responsibilities in your clinic would be most likely to fall under your auspices?
    a. Post-surgical patient safety
    b. Medical equipment maintenance
    c. Health record integrity
    d. Financial asset security

52. Patient satisfaction surveys have recently revealed customer service challenges at Hospital A across multiple departments. What important element should be considered when building a performance improvement team to handle this issue?
    a. The team should carefully evaluate patient feedback on customer service.
    b. The team should be assembled with members from every affected department.
    c. The team should establish clear goals and benchmarks for future feedback.
    d. All of the above

53. As a new administrator, you are eager to address some issues you have seen and improve the efficiency of various departments. But as you begin to implement changes, you encounter a great deal of resistance from staff members. What would be the best first step in understanding this resistance and making appropriate and effective changes?
   a. Understanding the history and culture of the organization
   b. Providing training classes and seminars about the changes
   c. Implementing punishment for those uncooperative with the changes
   d. Refraining from making any changes for at least a year

54. Which of the following is an example of qualitative data collection?
   a. Reviewing post-surgical infection statistics
   b. Surveying patients for satisfaction levels
   c. Analyzing employee attendance rates
   d. Collecting emergency room wait-time data

55. As part of an initiative for administrators to be more involved in day-to-day business, you have been spending a great deal of time in the wards of Hospital B. You notice there seem to be unreasonably long wait times between patient requests and nurse responses. What statistical process could you use to determine if this is a new or worsening problem?
   a. Random variation
   b. Qualitative data collection
   c. Trend analysis
   d. Special cause variation

56. When evaluating data for length of stay after cholecystectomy, you discover a very large standard deviation in the data. What could account for this?
   a. Diverse provider preferences for post-surgical length of stay
   b. Diverse post-surgical needs of cholecystectomy patients
   c. An error in calculation of the mean
   d. A and B

57. You are the administrator of a growing hospital, and you are considering applying for the Malcolm Baldrige National Quality Award for your organization. As you weigh the costs in time and money against the benefits of application, which benefit would most likely be the strongest encouragement for application?
   a. The notoriety of the award
   b. The rigors of self-assessment
   c. The value of site-visit feedback
   d. The government ties to the program

58. As a performance improvement team facilitator, what are your most important functions?
   a. Motivating and communicating effectively
   b. Allocating resources and mining data
   c. Instructing and redirecting employees
   d. Dictating duties and reprimanding offenders

59. Which of the following is a valid role on a performance improvement team?
    a. Team leader
    b. Team member
    c. Team facilitator
    d. All of the above

60. What is the most important first step of an effective performance improvement team?
    a. Make changes to organizational practices
    b. Evaluate the effectiveness of implemented change
    c. Identify a specific process that needs improvement
    d. Educate employees on changes to be made

61. After three wrong-site surgeries in one year, Hospital A determined a need to change preoperative practices to help eliminate this issue. Their best response would be...
    a. Suggesting surgeons double check patient charts prior to surgery.
    b. Firing and replacing all involved surgical staff and support personnel.
    c. Creating written procedures mandating better preoperative communication.
    d. Highlighting surgical notes in patient charts for easier access.

62. Although patient safety events are occurring with unacceptable frequency within your organization, staff members are reluctant to report these events because they fear retribution. What can be done to improve staff reporting?
    a. Nothing will improve staff reporting
    b. Implement a non-punitive reporting policy
    c. Increase punishments for reporting
    d. Implement punishment for not reporting

63. What effect will an extreme organizational focus on financial report results likely have on patient safety?
    a. It will have no effect on patient safety
    b. It will have a positive effect on patient safety
    c. It will have a negative effect on patient safety
    d. It will complicate patient safety policies

64. Who is responsible for patient safety in a healthcare organization?
    a. The patient safety officer
    b. Administrators and managers
    c. A and B
    d. All members of an organization

65. What is the management term for a comprehensive expression of an organization's identity and purpose?
    a. Vision statement
    b. Mission statement
    c. Cultural statement
    d. Organizational statement

66. Using Donabedian's model, which of the following areas most needs to be addressed in a clinic with elevated levels of post-treatment infection?
   a. Structure measures
   b. Process measures
   c. Outcome measures
   d. None of the above

67. A recent article from a prestigious health ranking organization has placed Hospital A at the very bottom of a list of regional hospitals. In order to move up in the rankings, what should Hospital A do first?
   a. Establish a steering committee to pinpoint problems and identify solutions
   b. Replace individuals at the administrative level with new hires
   c. Establish a quality council to enforce quality standards
   d. Launch an extensive public relations campaign to improve image

68. National mortality rates for heart attack victims have recently come across your desk. If you want to conduct a one-sample t-test comparing mortality rates at your hospital with national rates, what should your first step be?
   a. Find the standard deviation for the national heart attack mortality rates
   b. Gather mortality rates for a random sample of heart attack patients at your hospital
   c. Do a direct comparison of heart attack mortality variance rates at your hospital
   d. Collect qualitative data on heart attack mortality

69. You have established a patient satisfaction benchmark of 90 percent for each individual provider in your department. One provider consistently has scores between 87 and 89 percent over the course of a year. How would you describe his performance against the benchmark?
   a. Slightly substandard
   b. Dramatically substandard
   c. Standard
   d. Above standard

70. It has recently been brought to your attention that there is a disparity in admission rates between insured and uninsured patients with the same conditions. How could you best express this disparity statistically?
   a. Through use of a Pareto chart
   b. By using benchmark data
   c. Through comparative analysis
   d. By evaluating standard deviation

71. After three years of rising influenza rates, Clinic A institutes an extensive vaccination campaign. What outcome data would be expected as a result of this campaign?
   a. More clinic visitors
   b. Higher healthcare costs
   c. Reduced clinic visits
   d. Decreased influenza incidence

72. Which of the following are important areas to consider when evaluating a public health surveillance system for data collection?
    a. Data quality
    b. System experience
    c. Validity of acquired data
    d. All of the above

73. Hospital A has just implemented a new electronic health record system. As an administrator, it is your job to get everyone comfortable using this new system. What would be the best first step in this process?
    a. Presenting system benefits to stakeholders
    b. Requiring mandatory training for all employees
    c. Requiring mandatory usage by all employees
    d. Distributing a list of other organizations using the technology

74. When does the credentialing process generally take place?
    a. Prior to employment
    b. Prior to termination
    c. Every year of employment
    d. Every five years of employment

75. As a member of a quality improvement team, you are participating in a medication usage review. Who else must participate in this process?
    a. The patient
    b. A care provider
    c. A and B
    d. None of the above

76. Patients on the post-surgical ward have been complaining about a lack of privacy when nurses are performing wound care. What process is most appropriate to initiate for resolution of this issue?
    a. Quality control
    b. Patient advocacy
    c. Quality assurance
    d. Peer review

77. It is confirmed that a patient who sat for 30 minutes in the waiting room of your clinic was diagnosed with measles. What necessary infection-control step should be taken?
    a. Educate the patient on possible effects of the measles
    b. Document the case in your annual clinic statistics
    c. Train front-desk employees to recognize signs of measles
    d. Contact all patients who may have been in the waiting room that day

78. You have been tasked with creating patient safety training for the nursing staff. What is your first step in preparing training materials?
    a. Determine learning objectives
    b. Write lessons for presentation
    c. Create supplemental materials
    d. Schedule training times/locations

79. Which of the following are efficient ways to evaluate the effectiveness of performance improvement training?
    a. Exit surveys for participants
    b. Analysis of post-training performance
    c. Post-training focus groups with participants
    d. All of the above

80. When providing customer service training to employees from multiple departments, what is the most important concept to keep in mind?
    a. Diverse scheduling needs
    b. Lack of familiarity among trainees
    c. How differences may affect learning
    d. Some employees may not need training

81. What is the primary purpose and ultimate goal of performance improvement training?
    a. To improve performance in a specific area
    b. To improve performance throughout an organization
    c. To introduce new ideas to employees
    d. To create uniformity across an organization

82. Who can initiate a peer review?
    a. A patient
    b. A physician
    c. An insurance carrier
    d. All of the above

83. What is the relationship between peer review and root cause analysis?
    a. They are unrelated
    b. Peer review sparks root cause analysis
    c. They work together in failure analysis
    d. They were both designed by the Joint Commission

84. You are deeply involved in preparing an award application, and you need to survey internal subject matter experts to answer the questions needed for the application. What question would be appropriate for any survey, regardless of the department or subject?
    a. Describe your departmental approach to patient care
    b. Describe your departmental approach to customer service
    c. Describe your departmental approach to financial management
    d. All of the above

85. Which regulatory body is responsible for the Hospital Consumer Assessment of Healthcare Providers and Systems (HCAHPS) currently in use in more than 98 percent of acute care hospitals?
    a. The Joint Commission
    b. The Centers for Medicare and Medicaid Services (CMS)
    c. The Agency for Healthcare Research and Quality (AHRQ)
    d. B and C

86. Which of the following methods would be most appropriate for discussing individual patient management issues with a care provider?
   a. One-on-one discussion
   b. Focus group
   c. Care provider survey
   d. All of the above

87. How should quality management within a healthcare organization be viewed?
   a. As an event
   b. As a burden
   c. As a continuum
   d. As a finite process

88. As a department manager, you are trying to establish provider response time benchmarks. The data that you receive is aggregated data outlining all provider activities for your department. What should your first step be in working toward establishing benchmarks?
   a. Ask for a re-mining of data
   b. De-aggregate and classify data
   c. Establish only broad benchmarks
   d. Distribute data to employees

89. Which of the following might have a place on an individual performance improvement report?
   a. Time on job
   b. Gender
   c. Age
   d. None of the above

90. As an administrator, you are planning to implement a process change that will improve patient safety throughout your organization. Who will likely play the biggest role in getting employees motivated to change?
   a. Champions
   b. Administrators
   c. New hires
   d. Team facilitators

91. While reviewing year-end statistics, you notice your hospital performs many more tonsillectomies than other hospitals in the area. What response would be most appropriate to determine the cause of this statistical anomaly?
   a. Peer review
   b. Awards to providers
   c. Patient advocacy
   d. Medical record review

92. Despite repeated training, the emergency room staff still exceeds suggested organizational wait times for incoming patients. What factor should be considered before future training to ensure change will occur?
   a. Misalignment of departmental and organizational strategic goals
   b. Age and generational differences of department employees
   c. Gender-based bias of treatment times for incoming patients
   d. Standard deviation of staffing levels against patient influx levels

93. What provides the foundation for a performance improvement project?
    a. The budget
    b. The personnel involved
    c. The desired outcome
    d. The process for improvement

94. Hospital B has seen a recent increase in post-surgical wound infections. Investigation of the problem reveals a recurring issue with proper wound care by several members of the nursing staff. What would be the best departmental approach to this issue?
    a. Root cause analysis
    b. Punishment of involved staff members
    c. Implementation of a performance improvement team
    d. Utilization management assessment

95. Which of the following is the best definition of "champions"?
    a. High performers from various departments
    b. Credible and influential staff members
    c. Well-educated and highly-trained professionals
    d. Employees with long tenure at the organization

96. Employees are reducing your productivity by continually coming into your office with complaints and questions. As a manager, you want employees to address these issues with their direct supervisors. Then the supervisors can come to you with any questions. How can you best establish this structure?
    a. Reduce your office hours
    b. Reverse your open-door policy
    c. Train supervisors in assertiveness
    d. Clearly define lines of authority

97. You are part of a cost-analysis team evaluating a proposed inpatient nutrition program. What is the first step your team should take in the cost analysis process?
    a. Study framing
    b. Report formatting
    c. Audience defining
    d. Patient polling

98. Hospital A is preparing for international accreditation. As an administrator, what should you do to help prepare for the accreditation process?
    a. Prepare staff for the procedures of the process
    b. Compile all documents necessary for accreditation
    c. Ensure each department meets current standards
    d. All of the above

99. Which of the following is defined as correction of faulty processes to improve the quality of outcomes?
    a. Six Sigma
    b. Peer review
    c. Quality improvement
    d. None of the above

100. As an administrator faced with mounting surgical errors and complications, you are determined to improve the situation. Which of the following would be the most appropriate step toward operating room quality improvement?
    a. Enforcing pre-surgical full-team briefings
    b. Punishing surgeons involved in errors
    c. Scheduling surgeries later in the day
    d. Merging surgical and anesthesia teams

101. The pathology department of Hospital A is up for a service-specific review. What documents should be considered as part of this review?
    a. General policies and procedures for the hospital
    b. Employee work history and performance statistics
    c. Specific policies and procedures for pathology
    d. All of the above

102. What are some of the pitfalls faced when evaluating team performance?
    a. It is time-consuming and lacks objectivity.
    b. It is pointless and nonspecific.
    c. It is discriminatory and stressful.
    d. It is legally complex and doesn't improve productivity.

103. What tool is most effective in evaluating team performance?
    a. Focus groups
    b. Data mining
    c. Department meetings
    d. Anonymous surveys

104. When a hospital is facing low customer satisfaction ratings, what is the best initial goal in analyzing the data?
    a. Bring in experts to help analyze
    b. Identify the underlying problem
    c. Require mandatory training
    d. Re-survey dissatisfied customers

105. What is data inventory listing?
    a. Preparing a list of all reports currently produced
    b. Creating a spreadsheet that holds all available data
    c. Determining what information is available from which sources
    d. Taking inventory of all historical and organizational data

106. Which of the following chart types would be most effective in showing reduction of influenza incidence over time as a result of a vaccination program?
    a. Pareto chart
    b. Run chart
    c. Fishbone diagram
    d. Flow chart

107. Patient-safety incident reports at Hospital A have increased over the past two years by almost 20 percent according to recent data. Patient complaints have not increased significantly over this period. What is the most likely explanation for this trend?
   a. Patients are not noticing the incidents
   b. Incidents have actually increased by 20 percent
   c. Care providers are self-reporting incidents more
   d. None of the above

108. When disseminating health information to minority populations, which of the following considerations is most vital in ensuring efficacy?
   a. Timeliness
   b. Cultural appropriateness
   c. Entertainment value
   d. Educational content

109. Performance improvement results should be disseminated to employees primarily for the purpose of...
   a. Positive reinforcement.
   b. Departmental bragging rights.
   c. Educational motivation.
   d. Punishment of low performers.

110. What type of chart is most effective in demonstrating cause and effect?
   a. Flowchart
   b. Run chart
   c. Fishbone diagram
   d. Pareto chart

111. Which of the following is not likely to be included in a practitioner profile?
   a. Education and training
   b. Liability claims filed
   c. Staff/faculty privileges
   d. Practitioner age

112. The maternity ward of Hospital A has just added four FTE nursing staff members. After 60 days, productivity numbers do not seem to be increasing as expected. What is the most likely cause of this phenomenon?
   a. The learning curve for new employees
   b. An increase in patient needs
   c. A data reporting error
   d. Resentment of new staff by older employees

113. Clinic A has just completed six months of customer satisfaction surveys. Excellence in performance has been appropriately recognized. Now complaints must be analyzed and somehow quantified. What method would be most effective in the complaint analysis process?
   a. Sort surveys into separate folders
   b. Create a taxonomy for coding complaints
   c. Address complaints one at a time
   d. Match complaints with performance issues

114. As department manager, it is your job to conduct an annual performance appraisal for each employee in your department. One of your employees is exhibiting significant issues in response times for patient requests. How can you best incorporate performance improvement into the employee's performance appraisal?
    a. Incorporate punitive measures into the evaluation
    b. Use encouraging words to help the employee improve
    c. Set specific performance goals and a re-appraisal date
    d. Performance improvement is not part of performance appraisal

115. Which of the following are important elements of a written patient safety plan?
    a. Scope
    b. Purpose
    c. Guidelines
    d. All of the above

116. A seven-year-old girl receiving treatment for pneumonia at Hospital B has just been abducted by her non-custodial parent. Under standard patient safety guidelines, how would this event be classified?
    a. As an adverse incident
    b. As a sentinel event
    c. As a Baldrige occurrence
    d. As a risk management anomaly

117. What is the primary purpose of a patient safety program?
    a. To reduce medical errors and hazards
    b. To comply with local and national standards
    c. To reduce liability and tort claims
    d. To meet accreditation requirements

118. Your clinic has had three recent instances of chart mix-ups. In each case, doctors made initial patient contact with the wrong chart in hand and incorrect information. What technology would be most helpful in this situation?
    a. Medication barcode scanners
    b. Tablet computers or smart phones
    c. Electronic health record software
    d. Individual record RFID tags

119. To ensure proper identification of transfusion patients, your organization has recently adopted a two-person bedside/chair-side verification process. What is this an example of?
    a. Requirements for accreditation
    b. National patient safety goals
    c. Joint Commission best practices
    d. Local and regional healthcare laws

120. After experiencing a sentinel event, Hospital A is required to perform a root cause analysis. Which of the following is not a requirement of a root cause analysis?
    a. It must be conducted as soon as possible after the event.
    b. All personnel involved in the event must be present.
    c. Legal affidavits must be taken before questioning.
    d. Blame and liability should not be discussed or assigned.

121. What role does performance improvement data play in the appointment/privilege delineation process?
    a. Performance improvement and appointment/privilege delineation are unrelated.
    b. Performance improvement should be required for appointment/privilege eligibility.
    c. Performance improvement should take place after appointment/privilege delineation.
    d. Performance improvement oversight should be the job of a newly-advanced employee.

122. A recent risk management assessment has demonstrated that several frequently-used pieces of medical equipment have not been serviced recently, posing a threat to proper patient care. What performance improvement process should be undertaken to correct this issue?
    a. Post/publish equipment maintenance guidelines
    b. Post/publish a set equipment maintenance schedule
    c. Designate a specific employee/group to oversee maintenance
    d. All of the above

123. How does performance improvement relate to risk management assessment?
    a. Performance improvement and risk management assessment are unrelated.
    b. Performance improvement is a part of risk management assessment.
    c. Risk management assessment is a part of performance improvement.
    d. Performance improvement corrects issues identified in risk management assessment.

124. Hospital A recently implemented shorter inpatient stays for most surgical procedures. A utilization management assessment has revealed, however, that more patients are returning to the emergency room for post-surgical treatment. What performance improvement measure would be most likely to reduce the incidence of post-surgical patient returns?
    a. Implement better pre-discharge evaluations
    b. Reverse the shorter-stay policies
    c. Provide more painkillers at discharge
    d. Carefully analyze the patient return data

125. Which of the following is an external quality review that measures compliance against an industry standard for healthcare organizations?
    a. Peer review
    b. Accreditation
    c. Root cause analysis
    d. Credentialing

Answers and Explanations

1. B: In the creation of an organizational vision statement, vision is a description—realistic or not—of an ideal future state. This description of an ideal future state gives shape to the goals of an organization. A vision statement does not involve detailed descriptions about the specific actions necessary for bringing the vision to fruition.

2. A: Decision criteria is a decision-making model that explores all options equally and gives unorthodox or unpopular options a fair chance, even when they are under dispute. Consensus is not the best choice because this approach often reduces decisions to options that everyone likes and discounts the unorthodox or unpopular options that could be appropriate and viable.

3. D: Comparative data would prove most helpful in improving the processes at St. Joseph's Hospital. By comparing their data and processes with those of higher-ranked medical facilities, process improvement solutions could be derived. A and B are incorrect because internal data, whether historical or contemporary, will not help identify the reasons for the last place ranking and will not help improve processes. C is wrong because quality control data is another internal measure that will only compare the existing processes with established internal standards.

4. B: An organization is a structure that is designed to bring a group together for the pursuit of specific goals and objectives. While management and delegation are both important, they are not central to the unification of a team or group for goal pursuit. They are aspects of the structure, but not the structure itself.

5. D: Mrs. Jones' evaluation of the medical office was based entirely on her patient care experience, not the actual quality of the office or staff.

6. A: When managers do not make conscious organizational decisions, those decisions are made by default according to circumstances. Decision making becomes reactive instead of pro-active, and more and more resources are devoted to managing current problems which could have been prevented, instead of planning for the future. This can lead to the beginning of a negative feedback loop which can be very destructive to an organization.

7. C: Quality assurance is a focus on outputs or quality after the point of production, including any corrective actions necessary to optimize post-production quality, as in the surgery performed to remove the implement left in the patient. A, B, and D are incorrect because they refer to quality processes that take place on different levels and are not corrective in the way that quality assurance is.

8. D: All of the statements presented in A, B, and C are true statements about quality in healthcare.

9. A: Competent management is not considered a principle of total quality. Customer focus, continuous improvement, and teamwork are the three principles of total quality.

10. C: Healthcare organizations are often classified as systems because they are a collection of parts that function as an interdependent whole.

11. B: System thinking that prescribes preventative actions to help prevent an impending problem is called preemptive medicine.

12. D: The World Health Organization Surgical Safety Checklist leads to tight coupling in the operating room by closely aligning the various individuals involved in the surgical process.

13. B: The Joint Commission set the standard that hospitals are responsible for health information security and integrity.

14. D: The best way to understand exactly what is happening in the intensive care unit (ICU) is to unbundle or disaggregate the data and analyze it again, looking for specific challenges with RN sick days.

15. C: Risk management is defined as taking steps to avoid and control risks within an environment to accomplish a desired outcome, and the hand washing policy helps manage the risk of infection.

16. A: The downside of a heavy data focus can be tunnel vision by managers, which can lead to oversight of non-measured errors.

17. C: An employee with experience in the field who has emotional intelligence (demonstrated by mentoring new hires) and a quest for new knowledge shows excellent leadership potential.

18. B: A physical therapy department assistant is an internal customer because he or she works within the organizational structure. The other choices all represent external customers.

19. D: Patients, internal customers, and stakeholders should all be considered when developing process requirements within a healthcare organization.

20. B: When a Joint Commission-accredited hospital experiences a sentinel event, a root cause analysis is performed.

21. A: When undertaking a goal-setting process, the best first step is to develop an overall picture of the smaller partial goals to be achieved. B is wrong because it disregards the overall goal for the sake of a single smaller goal. C and D are incorrect because they are reactive steps, not proactive steps.

22. D: If a strict time limit is established, all of these will occur - ER nurses will be overstressed, mistakes are likely to be made, and triage will be less thorough.

23. B: A balanced scorecard is a set of data that give a quick and comprehensive overview of performance. Process measurement is lengthy and generally focused on a single process area, not quick and all-encompassing. Dashboard scoring is not as quick or comprehensive as a balanced scorecard. Six Sigma deals with quality measurement, not performance data.

24. A: Epidemiological theory is used to identify the source and cause of an issue or anomaly, which is perfect for the surgical complications represented in this question.

25. C: The primary purpose of the Consumer Assessment of Health Providers and Systems (CAHPS) is to capture patient satisfaction data in a universal way that can be compared among all hospitals.

A, B, and D represent secondary or tertiary purposes of CAHPS; they do not represent its primary purpose.

26. D: It is vital that quality council members take external standards (such as national goals and requirements) into account when addressing the rising infection rates.

27. B: When data are aggregated, one of the biggest challenges is the loss of context, which makes specific solutions hard to identify.

28. B: When preparing the report on postpartum care to be presented to administrators, the most important goal is identifying which data are most relevant to the situation. A, C, and D are incorrect because while they may offer some items of interest, they do not best help you describe the situation at hand to the administration.

29. D: Surveys, focus groups, and informal discussions are all excellent ways to assess customer needs and expectations.

30. A: When healthcare data is transparent and visible to a number of populations, it encourages performance improvement to create more positive data, thereby improving the image of the organization. B and C are incorrect because while they may be true for some organizations, they do not represent the most important regulatory function of healthcare transparency.

31. C: The first priority in process improvement should be identifying the existing process issues. A, B, and D are incorrect because while they are good steps in the process improvement journey, they are not the first priority in the process.

32. A: Researching the causes of an employee's challenges has no place in the performance improvement plan process. A clear problem statement, specific action steps, and a goal behavior are all important elements in creating a performance improvement plan.

33. B: Clinical guidelines dictate process requirements for an organization, as new processes must fall into line with the guidelines of an organization and industry practices. A and D are incorrect because they minimize the relationship between clinical guidelines and process requirements. C is wrong because process requirements are governed by clinical guidelines, not the other way around.

34. A: When improving the patient safety culture, both patient perceptions and clinical quality must be taken into account and balanced.

35. C: Improving the effectiveness of caregiver communication is a patient safety goal that has been established by the Joint Commission. A, B, and D may be good goals, but they have not been established as specific patient safety goals by the Joint Commission.

36. B: An implicit goal of service time reduction is a potential adversary to patient safety because providers who are hurrying may not communicate effectively with patients.

37. D: A good patient survey will address the physical, emotional, and social needs of the patient to give a provider a complete picture of how the patient's needs can best be met.

38. A: The biggest benefit of Six Sigma is the goal of driving errors to zero, thereby dramatically improving the quality of care.

39. C: The most influential reason for implementing CPOE is the fact that it has been shown to reduce prescribing errors by 50 percent or more, thereby improving quality of care. A, B, and D may all be influencing reasons for adopting CPOE, but they should not be the deciding factor, as they are much less important than reducing prescribing errors.

40. C: Either a fishbone diagram or Pareto chart is the best way to visually represent a specific problem and a list of contributory causes. A and B are not correct because flowcharts, deployment charts, pie charts, and run charts are designed to present a variety of data, not just to illustrate a specific problem and its causes.

41. B: A root cause analysis is designed to investigate and pose possible remedies for a significant negative effect in a healthcare setting. A and C are not correct because they are both forward-looking evaluations instead of backward-looking investigations. D is wrong because it is not a relevant type of data analysis.

42. D: Process requirements are the element of process performance that represents the voice of the customer, outlining the change or action that is needed. A, B, and C are incorrect because although they are all elements of process performance, they are not the elements that help define the needed change or best course of action.

43. A: Benchmark data are valuable to the performance improvement process because they provide a comparison standard for behavior. B, C, and D are not the best choices because they do not demonstrate the way benchmark data can be used to help performance improvement.

44. C: The leader of a performance improvement team must model target behaviors above all else in order to set the example for team members.

45. D: The Joint Commission created the National Patient Safety Goals (NPSGs) to improve patient safety nationwide.

46. B: Implementing barcode medication administration technology is the most effective and efficient way to reduce errors in medication administration, as it uses technology to double-check work performed by nursing staff before the medication is actually administered. A, C, and D are incorrect because, while they may help correct the issue, they would take longer and be less reliable than barcode medication administration technology.

47. C: New customers often result from performance improvement initiatives, boosting an organization's bottom line.

48. D: A good manager will use satisfaction surveys, feedback forums, and careful data analysis to help identify the cause of the CNA issues and help reestablish the status quo.

49. C: Using an electronic medical record (EMR) keeps all patient information in a centralized location, making it easy to access and analyze.

50. A: Integrating new patient safety measures into existing strategic goals makes them easier to implement because of the level of familiarity with the current strategic goals.

51. C: The information technology department participates in risk management, with their area of expertise being health record integrity.

52. D: Carefully evaluating feedback, drawing members from multiple departments, and establishing clear future goals are all important elements of building a performance improvement team to resolve customer service issues.

53. A: The most important first step for a new administrator who wants to make changes is to understand the organizational history and culture and make changes appropriately.

54. B: Surveying patients is the only answer that results in qualitative feedback because the answers are more subjective and perspective-dependent than quantitative data. A, C, and D are incorrect because they produce quantitative data that is objective and not qualitative in nature.

55. C: Performing a trend analysis will reveal any changes in wait times over a set period of time, as well as any new or worsening problems. A, B, and D are wrong because, while they offer statistical analysis, they do not demonstrate long-term trends or changes in service levels.

56. D: Both diverse provider preferences and diverse patient needs could result in the dramatic standard deviation in the statistics. C is incorrect because a calculation error in determining the mean is not generally a reason for a significant standard deviation.

57. C: The potential value of site-visit feedback that can come as a result of applying for a Baldrige Award is the most encouraging factor for application.

58. A: The most important functions of a performance improvement team facilitator are motivation and communication. B, C, and D are not the best choices because, while a team facilitator may perform these duties, they are not the most important or even necessary functions of the team facilitator.

59. D: A performance improvement team is made up of a team leader, a team facilitator, and team members.

60. C: The most important first step for a performance improvement team is identifying a specific process that needs improvement.

61. C: Creating written policies mandating better pre-surgical communication would be the best response to the errors.

62. B: Implementing a non-punitive reporting policy is the best option to help encourage employees to report potential patient safety events. A is not the best choice because it represents capitulation to the problem instead of resolution. C and D are incorrect because increasing the punishments for voluntary reporters will discourage employees from reporting issues.

63. C: A strong organizational focus on financial report results, the so-called "bottom line," will likely have a negative effect on patient safety as efforts are made to lower costs of service.

64. D: All members of an organization, no matter their title or job duties, are responsible for patient safety.

65. B: A mission statement is a comprehensive expression of an organization's identity and purpose.

66. C: Outcome measures deal with the effects of treatment after the fact, so they are the most applicable portion of Donabedian's model to this particular situation. A and B are wrong because structure and process measures do not apply to this situation. D is incorrect because Donabedian's outcome measures do apply to this case.

67. A: To fix the low placement in rankings, Hospital A needs to establish a steering committee to pinpoint problem areas and identify potential solutions.

68. B: A one-sample t-test requires a random sample of applicable data, so gathering the random sample would be the first step in conducting the t-test. A, C, and D are incorrect because they do not fit into the framework of a one-sample t-test.

69. A: When a benchmark of 90 percent patient satisfaction has been set, a provider who consistently scored between 87 and 89 percent would have performance that was considered slightly substandard.

70. C: The best way to statistically express a disparity between two categories of data is through comparative analysis. A, B, and D are incorrect because, while they statistically express data, they do not show disparities within a data set and they do not compare numbers as clearly as comparative analysis does.

71. D: The expected result of the vaccination campaign by Clinic A would be decreased influenza incidence.

72. D: Data quality, system experience, and validity of acquired data are all important areas to consider when evaluating a public health surveillance system for data collection. A, B, and C are not correct because none of those options alone is the best answer, although they are all important elements of an effective system as a whole.

73. A: When implementing a new system and trying to get employees comfortable with it, one of the best first steps is presenting actual system benefits to stakeholders who can get others excited about the technology. B, C, and D are incorrect because although they are all possible tactics to get employees to use the new system, they are not effective as a first step.

74. A: Credentialing generally takes place prior to employment.

75. C: Both a patient and provider should be involved in a medication usage review to improve efficacy.

76. B: A lack of privacy during wound care should be resolved through the support of a patient advocate.

77. D: The most important infection-control step in this situation would be to contact all patients who may have been in the waiting room that day.

78. A: The first step in creating patient safety training (or any other kind of training) should be determining the learning objectives. B, C, and D are incorrect because, although they are valid steps in creating training, they do not represent the first step of the process.

79. D: Exit surveys for participants, analysis of post-training performance, and post-training focus groups are all effective ways to evaluate the effectiveness of performance improvement training.

80. C: The most important thing to keep in mind when providing customer service training for employees from multiple departments is how differences may affect learning.

81. A: The primary purpose and ultimate goal of performance improvement training is to improve performance in a specific area. B is incorrect because performance improvement should be targeted at a specific behavior to be improved. C and D wrong because, while they are both desirable goals, neither one represents the primary purpose and ultimate goal of performance improvement training.

82. D: A peer review may be initiated by a patient, a physician, or an insurance carrier.

83. C: Peer review and root cause analysis are both tools that are used hand-in-hand as part of failure analysis.

84. B: Every department can and should answer survey questions describing their approach to customer service.

85. D: The Hospital Consumer Assessment of Healthcare Providers and Systems (HCAHPS) was designed jointly by the Centers for Medicare and Medicaid Services (CMS) and the Agency for Healthcare Research and Quality (AHRQ).

86. A: One-on-one discussion is the best and most appropriate form of communication when discussing the management of an individual patient with a care provider.

87. C: Quality management of a healthcare organization should be viewed as a continuum that is always progressing toward the best possible outcomes.

88. B: De-aggregating and classifying data is the best first step in breaking down the aggregated data to determine specific data on provider response time.

89. A: Time on job might have a place on an individual performance improvement report because a new employee would not be expected to improve as quickly as an established employee, and an established employee should show improvement over their time on job.

90. A: Champions are respected "key players" in the organization and will therefore be most likely to play a big role in getting employees motivated to change.

91. D: In a statistical anomaly situation involving medical procedures, a medical record review would be warranted to determine why tonsillectomies were being performed more often than at other regional hospitals.

92. A: Before pursuing further training for the emergency room staff, it is important to examine if there is a misalignment of departmental goals (quality care) and organizational strategic goals (reduced wait times).

93. C: A specific desired outcome provides the foundation for a performance improvement project, serving as the target to be reached with improvements made.

94. C: When faced with recurring staff issues with wound care, implementing a performance improvement team is the best option, as it creates both a process and an incentive for improvement.

95. B: Champions are credible and influential staff members who can be very motivational in creating change.

96. D: As a manager, you must clearly define lines of authority to direct accountability where it belongs in the chain of command.

97. A: The first step in a standard cost analysis process is study framing. B and C are wrong because, although they are valid parts of cost analysis, they come later in the process, not as the first step. D is not correct because patient polling is not part of a standard cost analysis.

98. D: In preparation for international accreditation, administrators should prepare staff for the survey process, assist in compiling necessary documents, and ensure departments are meeting current standards.

99. C: Quality improvement is defined as correction of faulty processes to improve the quality of outcomes.

100. A: Enforcing pre-surgical full-team briefings would be the most appropriate step toward improving operating room quality in this situation.

101. C: A service-specific review of the pathology department would cover specific policies and procedures for pathology.

102. A: Some of the major pitfalls of team performance evaluations are the time they take and the lack of objectivity as team members evaluate one another.

103. D: Anonymous surveys are the most effective tool in evaluating team performance because they remove the fear of retribution for low rankings and a sense of obligation for high rankings.

104. B: When a hospital is facing low customer satisfaction ratings, the best first step is identifying the underlying problem, after which performance improvement can be coordinated. A, C, and D are incorrect because, while bringing in experts, requiring training, and re-surveying customers may happen later in the process, they are not good first steps.

105. C: Data inventory listing can be defined as determining what information is available from which sources, thereby making an inventory of available data sources.

106. B: A run chart is designed to show trending outcomes against passing time, which is perfect for the influenza incidence reduction presented in this question. A, C, and D are incorrect because even

though Pareto charts, fishbone diagrams, and flow charts are accurate ways to visually display information, they do not fit the parameters of the given situation.

107. C: Increased provider self-reporting is the most likely cause of the increased incident reporting in light of the absence of an increase in customer complaints.

108. B: When disseminating health information to minority populations, cultural appropriateness is the most important consideration for efficacy because culturally inappropriate presentations of information will likely be ignored.

109. A: The main effect of performance improvement results among employees is an overall sense of positive reinforcement that encourages them to maintain the good work. B, C, and D are incorrect because, while they represent possible effects of performance improvement results, they are not the primary purpose of dissemination of results to employees.

110. C: A fishbone diagram is the best type of visual representation to show cause and effect because it demonstrates how various effects branch from the same cause.

111. D: Practitioner age has no place in a practitioner profile, as it is irrelevant to competence levels, skills, and abilities. The other answer choices all represent information that belongs in a practitioner profile.

112. A: Productivity generally takes a brief dip after the addition of new employees due to the learning curve and their need for assistance from established staff members.

113. B: The most effective way to analyze large numbers of complaints is through the creation of a taxonomy for coding complaints because it helps classify and organize complaints in a logical way that lends itself well to analysis.

114. C: The best way to incorporate performance improvement concepts into an employee appraisal is through specific performance goals and a set re-appraisal date. A and B are incorrect because they are not concrete performance improvement techniques.

115. D: A written patient safety plan includes a scope, a purpose, and guidelines.

116. B: Abduction qualifies as a sentinel event under Joint Commission guidelines and standard practices.

117. A: The primary purpose of a patient safety program is to reduce medical errors and hazards.

118. C: Electronic health record software is the best choice for preventing paper chart mix-ups and to ensure that doctors meet the patient with the most accurate and up-to-date information possible.

119. B: Two-person bedside/chair-side verification of transfusion patients is a clear example of national patient safety goals being put into place.

120. C: During a root cause analysis, legal affidavits are not required before questioning. All of the other answer choices are elements that are required as part of a root cause analysis.

121. B: Performance improvement, as demonstrated over time with an organization, should be a required element for appointment/privilege delineation because it gives an idea of a provider's commitment to an organization and to quality.

122. D: As part of performance improvement on the equipment maintenance, guidelines should be published or posted, a maintenance schedule should be published or posted, and a specific employee or group should be designated to handle maintenance.

123. D: Performance improvement is related to risk management because it is a tool to correct the issues that are uncovered during a risk management assessment.

124. A: Implementing better pre-discharge evaluations is the most likely option for reducing post-surgical patient returns.

125. B: Accreditation is an external quality review that measures compliance against industry standards.